Where Does It Hurt?

Where Does It Hurt?

Further Adventures of a Country Vet

Dr. David Perrin

Illustrations by Wendy Liddle

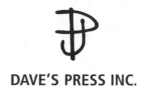

DAVE'S PRESS INC.

Published by Dave's Press Inc.
Box 616, Lister
British Columbia
Canada V0B 1Y0

Cover and book design by Warren Clark
Illustrations by Wendy Liddle
Edited by Betsy Brierley
Proofread by Elizabeth McLean

Printed and bound in Canada

National Library of Canada Cataloguing in Publication

Perrin, David, 1948–
    Where does it hurt? : further adventures of a country vet/
    David Perrin ; illustrated by Wendy Liddle.

    ISBN 0-9687943-2-7

    1. Perrin, David, 1948-. 2. Veterinarian—British
Columbia–Biography. 3. Animals—Anecdotes. I. Title.
SF613.P47A3 2003   636.089'092   C2003-906981-8

To the memory of
Swami Sivananda Radha

Acknowledgements

It seemed that this day would never come, but perseverance has finally coaxed *Where Does It Hurt?* into being. This book recounts a period of personal growth that occurred thirty years ago. Perhaps it was appropriate that as I was writing this third book, I again revisited the meaning of life and re-examined what is truly important.

There is no question that friends and family were what remained at the bottom of the pan after my search for the true "gold" of my existence. They rallied behind me to keep me from giving up. I offer my sincere thanks to my sisters, Kay Rizzotti and Audrey O'Hearn, for reminding me what family is all about. Thank you Joan, Marshall, Gordon, and Alicia for supporting your father through a difficult time. Thank you Todd Francoeur, John Gallagher, Gopalananda, Dan Hurford, Jim Karountzos, Darcie Rodgers, and Sean for teaching me the meaning of friendship.

I extend my thanks to Yasodhara Ashram and those dedicated individuals who have taken up Swami Radha's banner. May you keep the sanctuary alive and healthy for others who stumble along the path and need help to see the possibilities of the future. I offer my gratitude to the members of the Yoga Development Class of 2003 for sharing so much with me.

As with the first two books in the "Dr. Dave" series, my editor Betsy Brierley, my illustrator Wendy Liddle, my designer Warren Clark, and my proofreader Elizabeth McLean have helped bring *Where Does It Hurt?* to life. I couldn't ask for better support than they have provided.

The encouragement of my readers through e-mail and letters has been a great help in maintaining the momentum. Many times your words have buoyed my spirits and motivated me to keep on plowing that long furrow. May you find renewed enjoyment in my third collection of veterinary adventures.

Contents

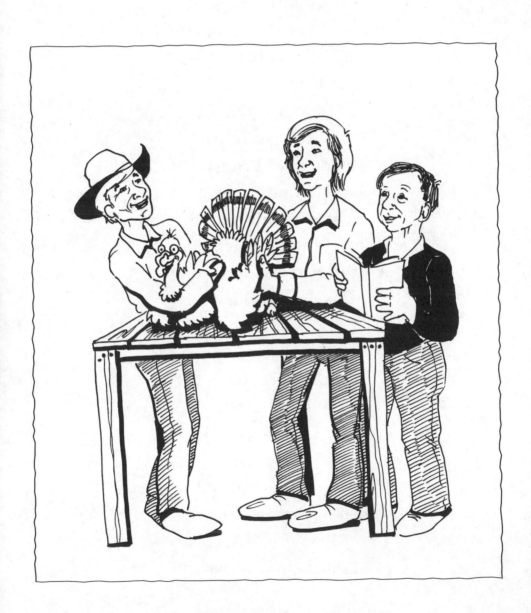

Gold Fingers

I reached over the brim of the pelvis, hooked my fingers under the cervix, and flipped the uterus backwards onto the pelvic floor. Gently manipulating the uterine wall, I worked the organ back and forth between my thumb and forefinger. The sensation of delicate membranes slipping between my fingers was unmistakeable.

"She's pregnant."

Jack Rodgers smiled. "Damn time...I've had the devil of a time catchin' her in heat. I was about ready to get myself a bull."

I removed my arm from the cow, turned the glove inside out, and quickly knotted it. As I ducked my head to avoid a rafter, Jack pointed to the cow's manger.

"What do you think of my incubator, Doc?" There sat a tiny hen with her head tucked tight to the corner. "She's the best thing you can imagine when it comes to hatchin' out chicks. I took away most of her own eggs last time and switched them with a bunch from a Rhode Island Red hen. She hatched and raised the whole mess of them."

"Bantams are amazing when it comes to maternal instincts," I agreed. The little brown and white bird seemed to sense that she had become the centre of attention and was doing her best to blend with the straw she was nesting on.

"Got her workin' on some turkey eggs now. She's been settin' them for ages. Do they take longer than hens' eggs? All of the Rhode Island chicks and a few of her own have hatched out. I've been watchin' like a hawk, but I haven't seen anything that would pass for a turkey."

"Have you candled any of the eggs to see if they're good?" I tapped the manure-filled plastic sleeve against my leg and took a step toward the door.

"What do you mean, candle them? This hobby farmin' gets more complicated by the minute."

"You hold an egg up to the light and look for evidence of the developing embryo inside."

Jack reached under the hen and removed a huge turkey egg that the surrogate mom had been incubating. Several chicks scattered at his intrusion, and the hen pecked aggressively at his fingers. "Show me. I've been dyin' to get some turkey chicks."

He handed me the egg, and I held it up to the bare light bulb in the centre of the barn. "Come look." I rotated the egg around and around. "See how the entire content appears to be a homogeneous mass?"

"Yeah," Jack affirmed.

"If there were a chick inside, you'd be able to make out its shadow through the shell."

"Well, I'll be darned. That means it's not good, then?" Jack had a hard time hiding his disappointment.

I cracked the egg on the side of a four-by-four upright and dumped a watery, foul-smelling liquid into the gutter.

"Damn it, anyway!" Jack cursed. "I bet the rest of 'em are the same."

He rousted the bird and handed me half a dozen eggs one after the other. They were all in similar condition. "I wonder why they all rotted?" He pushed back his cowboy hat, shook his head in disgust, and spoke to the distressed little hen. "You may as well forget it, girl…You're not goin' to get any more babies."

We left the barn and headed in the direction of the house. We hadn't gone more than a few paces when Jack turned on his heel and headed back.

"Take a quick look at these critters and see if you can see something wrong with them."

He took me to an enclosed yard where a few hens and a huge tom turkey rushed forward for the grain that he tossed on the ground in front of them.

"Don't they look in good shape to you?" Jack surveyed my face as I examined his birds.

They appeared to be in fine condition—especially the tom. He was simply massive. I watched as the huge grey bird spread his wings, fanned his tail, and paraded up and down in front of his flock. The sides of his head were so disgustingly red, his wattle so shockingly purple.

"You realize that in commercial flocks they breed all the hens artificially."

"Oh. Okay, so how do they do that?"

"Well, the usual," I answered. "They collect the tom's semen for insemination."

"Okay." Then the penny dropped. "Oh! They *collect* it."

I nodded. Jack gave me a look of incredulity. "It's bad enough tryin' to catch a cow in heat, let alone foolin' around with these critters." He shook his head and resumed his tirade. "I can see breeding the cows artificially so I don't have to keep a bull around, but why should the hens be bred artificial with this big sucker here?"

"It may well be that he's too big. When they get as heavy as he is, they sometimes can't even mount the hens properly."

Jack screwed up his face and looked at me intently. "You're not shittin' me, are you?"

"No, the problem is that they've bred these birds to be so big that they have trouble mounting and breeding. It's the same for a lot of the meat-bird chickens, too."

"I'll be damned…The only reason I kept those guys was to raise some of my own. Now it looks like I'd be just as far ahead to butcher them off and buy new chicks."

Several horses plodded along beside us as we returned to the house. Jack was sulking. He was obviously perturbed that his plan to rear his own turkeys was falling apart. I could understand completely how he felt. As a small producer, it was easy to get into the mode of wanting to do for oneself—there was nothing like being totally self-sufficient.

Jack opened the swinging gate by the house and we passed through. He had just lowered the hoop latch over the last rung on the gate when he turned to me with a look of determination.

"So, can you do it?"

"Uh…we went over it in an animal science class at the vet college," I replied. "I'm sure we'd be able to figure it out."

"Well, let's try. I want some chicks out of 'em."

Later that morning I dug through my reference material and was elated to find that my book on poultry management had a complete description of the technique for collecting semen from tom turkeys and the artificial insemination of the hen. After a quick read, I determined it sounded like something we could handle.

I called Jack and told him that with just a little bit of luck, we could probably pull off the operation. He was so excited at the prospect that he insisted we get at it right after lunch. Jack was a contractor and was working on a new home in Lister. The fact that he was supposed to be laying out the footings for the house took a back seat to this new venture. He was sure that the people wouldn't mind his slacking off so long as he showed up for a couple of hours after supper.

Before leaving the office I dug up a glass beaker, a dozen insulin syringes, some bowls, and my book on poultry production. I was certain that I had everything necessary to succeed at immaculate conception in turkeys.

When I got to the Rodgers' Canyon home, the drive was so plugged with vehicles that I had to park on the side of the road behind several other cars. I knew Sandy, Jack's wife, ran a hair salon from a basement office and frequently had customers—but this was something different.

I got out of my car and looked uncertainly up the roadway. We were at a dip in the road, and I began fretting about the possibility that someone might hit my car. Before I could worry too much, a vehicle pulled up behind me. A middle-aged woman with a wide-brimmed hat and a frilly summer dress hopped out, straightened herself, and rushed up the driveway.

I bustled along after her with my trusty stainless bucket in one arm and my box of supplies under the other. Waiting at the back gate was Jack with a man I had never seen before. Damn it all, anyway, I cursed under my breath. Jack knew this was a procedure I was uncertain about. Why in hell did he have someone else tagging along? It seemed as if I always had to perform a new act in front of an audience.

"Dave, I'd like you to meet Phil McGraw. He's bought a place out in Lister. We're just laying footings for his house."

The man stepped forward. "Glad to meet you."

"You'll have enough to keep you going over at his place," Jack chirped. "McGraw's got a regular zoo out there."

I handed Jack my bucket. "Let's not forget the warm water. We have to keep the semen from cooling off while we're getting ready for the hens."

While we waited for Jack to get back with the water, Phil filled me in on all his critters. He had a tremendous selection of pets—along with half a dozen horses—and he certainly sounded like a good potential for future business.

Jack was in a rush to get going. Water slopped from the pail as he approached at a half-run. He led us through the gate past a group of women. Several were seated around a picnic table with tall glasses in their hands, but others were relaxing on lawn chairs. They were engrossed in conversation—the result was the din of twenty women all talking at the same time.

"Sandy's havin' a bit of a hen party today," Jack commented sarcastically. "Something to do with her cosmetic sales. She had me mowin' lawns and pullin' weeds all morning to get ready for this darn thing."

Almost all of my concerns about an audience for this procedure were now manifest.

We proceeded to the turkey run with Jack and Phil making jokes about my magic fingers. Phil determined that once Old Tom had experienced Doc's "gold fingers," he'd be so enamoured with his big new buddy that Jack would have trouble keeping him home.

Jack threw out a handful of grain, and the birds jostled one another in a rush for their share. I opened my book and began reading over the procedure one more time. Jack was about to throw out more grain when I stopped him.

"It says here that the semen should be clear of fecal material, and that most producers will withhold feed and water from the tom for eight to twelve hours to help avoid contamination of the semen."

Jack hesitated as Old Tom strutted back and forth in front of him, raising and lowering his head in anticipation of more grain.

"So what d'ya have to do to get Tom to come across?" McGraw chortled. "Wander out in the pen, bend over, and start gobbling?"

Ignoring his barbs, I referred to the text. "It says here that semen may be collected from toms two or three times per week."

"That's a lot better than I'm doin'," Jack interjected.

I read on. "Milking or working a tom takes two people. One holds the bird on a padded table or his lap with the tail end of the bird toward the other operator."

"I got an old table in the barn," Jack interrupted. "I'll get it."

While Jack ran for the table, I read the description over and over, trying to determine whether we held Tom on his back or left him on his stomach. I turned the page and stared at the black and white photographs, trying to be certain as to the orientation. The tail feathers all seemed to be pointing straight up in the pictures. I watched Old Tom parading in front of his hens and tried to picture his holding still in either position. I was still uncertain when Jack plunked the table down in front of me.

"What next?"

I tossed the book, open to page 52, on the table. "How are they holding him…tummy down or tummy up?"

Jack and Phil knelt on the ground in front of the book. "He's tummy up," said Phil.

"He can't be!" argued Jack. "See! There are the tail feathers going up."

"Where's his head?" I asked.

Jack opened his mouth as if to answer, then hesitated.

"See," insisted Phil, "he's on his back!" He indicated the photo on page 53 and poked it emphatically with his index finger.

"But that picture's of them putting the tom's jizz in the hen," Jack countered. "See? It says right here it's when they're doing the insemination." Jack articulated the word insemination carefully.

I studied the pictures, trying to get my orientation. It was so confusing. For some reason, I had been absolutely certain that the tom would have to be positioned on his back. Now, I wasn't at all sure.

"I wonder why the guy who wrote this wouldn't have thought about mentioning which end is up?" Jack pondered.

"Probably because he doesn't think anyone would be fool enough to even think of doing it the other way," I replied.

"See…it says right here," McGraw interjected, "that one guy holds the bird with the tail end to the other operator." He read on: "The second person then stimulates the tom by stroking his abdomen and pushing the tail upward and toward the bird's head."

"Yeah, right," Jack declared. "And how can he do that if the bird is upside down?"

Phil screwed up his face and read the passage again. "Damned if I know…You may be right."

In the meantime, Tom continued circling around and around with his head held high and his wings outstretched, as if he knew that we were talking about him.

"When was the last time he was handled?" I asked Jack.

"Probably when he was a chick. The kids love fiddlin' with them when they're chicks. Since then he's gone everywhere under his own steam."

"You know, when we're handling parakeets and canaries, they tell us to cover them with a towel so they can't see—that way they struggle less. I brought one to throw over his head, but looking at the size of him, we may be better off with a blanket."

"Let me grab a saddle blanket," said Jack.

Phil and I climbed over the fence and herded the birds into a tight corner near their waterer. Most indignant about the goings on, Tom strutted back and forth, fanning his tail and gobbling in complaint. The closer I got to him, the more daunting seemed the task. He was a big boy. We'd have to get something over those wings to keep him from beating us half to death and to prevent his injuring himself.

He fixed his wings and extended his massive head. Gobbling aggressively, he wagged his huge purple wattle from side to side. Jack appeared on the other side of the fence, unfolding a large grey woollen blanket as he ran. His eyes were focused on Tom.

"Are we ready?" he asked.

"As ready as we're going to be," I replied.

He threw the blanket during one of Tom's displays of prowess. I dove in and held the gobbler's wings tight to his body. He struggled briefly, lifting first one leg, then the other in a desperate attempt to rake me with his spurs.

"Easy, fellow," I chimed. "Grab his legs, guys, and we'll get him in position."

Jack climbed over the fence to enter the fray. Snaring both of Tom's feet, he headed for the table.

"Get the book, Phil, and read us our instructions," I directed.

"Been a long time since McGraw needed written instructions for jerking off," Jack needled.

Tom struggled briefly when we lay his breast on the table, making a futile attempt at flapping his wings.

"Okay, boys, let's get this show on the road."

I immersed the beaker I had prepared for collection and the Baggie full of tuberculin syringes in the water. "It's important that the collection stuff is warm enough to keep from shocking the sperm cells."

McGraw picked up the book and perused the page. "It says to hold the legs slightly spread apart to expose the abdomen."

Jack opened up the distance between his hands and between Tom's legs.

"Then it says that the second person stimulates the tom by stroking its abdomen and pushing the tail up toward the head."

"By God, this is just like in the army days," Jack interjected. "There were guys payin' for treatment like this in the brothels back in Korea...Being tied up with a blanket over my head was never much of a turn-on for me, though."

"Some of us would never know, Jack," McGraw countered.

I began stroking the bird's abdomen, applying firm but gentle pressure toward the tail. Tom promptly shot a jet of juicy wet feces onto the toe of Jack's cowboy boot.

"Aw, Tom," Jack complained, "that's not what we're lookin' for." He lifted his foot, flicked it a few times, and wiped his boot on the back of his pant leg.

I stroked Tom again and pushed forward on his tail. His vent puckered several times, then relaxed.

"It says," McGraw read on, "when you push forward on his tail the male copulatory organ enlarges and partially protrudes from the vent."

"Come on, Tom," Jack prompted, "get it up for the doc."

Sure enough, when I pushed forward on his tail, a pink blob of flesh protruded.

McGraw continued with his instructions. "Now, it says the second person grips the rear of the copulatory organ with his thumb and forefinger from above and fully exposes the organ."

I pressed at the base of the blob and up popped the organ.

Phil continued reading. "It says to squeeze out the semen with a short, sliding, downward movement."

I positioned the beaker.

Phil could no longer contain himself. "Get ready, Tom—here comes Gold Fingers."

I closed my fingers around the organ and pulled down expectantly. Nothing happened.

"More pressure," suggested Jack.

I tried again.

"A bit faster," suggested Phil.

Same result. I began the procedure all over again, firmly stroking Tom's abdomen. I pushed his tail upward toward his head. Up popped the pink blob. This time the copulatory organ was enlarged and protruding from the vent. I squeezed forward on the organ, and four drops of milky fluid dripped into the beaker.

"That's it?" Jack asked glumly.

"Half a millilitre max is what the book claims."

"Jack!" Sandy's voice rang out from the backyard, where the garden party was in full swing. "Jack!"

"What the hell now?" Jack grumbled, setting the tom back on his feet. "Phil, can you give her a holler and tell her I'm tied up."

Phil retreated and a moment later we heard, "Yeah, Sandy?"

"Tell Jack that the builders' supply is on the line about your materials!" she answered. "They say it's important."

Phil's reply echoed throughout the neighbourhood. "He's all tied up and can't take the call right now! He and Doc Perrin are busy jacking off Tom."

Silence.

I cringed and glanced at Jack. "Does she have the faintest idea what we're up to?"

"Not from me, she doesn't," he replied. "Haven't talked to her since I left the house this morning—she's been so busy all day gettin' ready for this shindig."

"Oh my God…"

The party was still in full swing by the time we finished inseminating the hens with their tiny portion of semen. A few women giggled and waved as I skulked past them on my way to the car. Jack had done his level best to fill them in on what was really going on.

I laughed out loud. Marcie would have seen the humour in this situation.

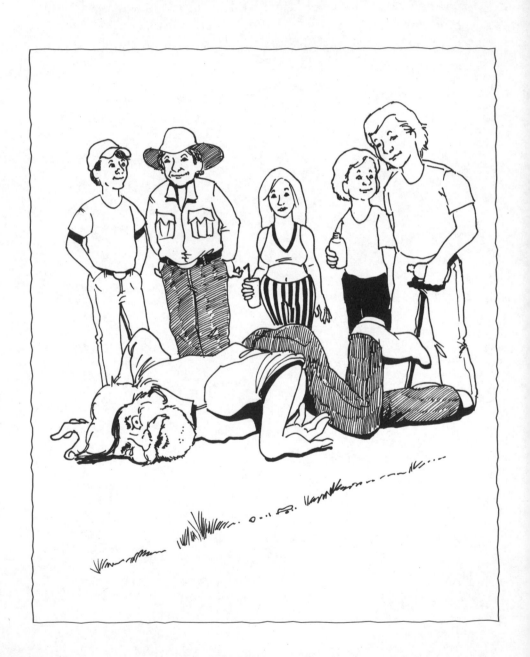

Fist Fight at the Yahk Hotel

There seemed to be no end to the unusual situations a veterinarian could find himself in—especially here in the Kootenays. I chuckled, thinking back to the latest adventure—the Yahk Raft Race. As gruelling as the experience had been, I was glad I had entered. Marcie had been a real trooper during the race. In hindsight, I couldn't have chosen a better partner.

We had just been plucked from the icy waters of the Moyie. Cory, Marcie, Barb, and I were now survivors of the infamous river challenge, having successfully completed the two-hour journey down ten miles of fast-running current on a homemade cedar-log barge. What was even more miraculous, Marcie and I had lost our own raft and navigated the last few miles on a craft that we found flipped upside down and abandoned in a back eddy. The event had tested us dearly.

Shivering, I closed my eyes and pulled the woollen blanket closer to my body. Wet denim clung to my legs like a lead weight. Water squished between my toes as I shifted uneasily from one foot to the other. Although my fingers were regaining some sensation, I still had difficulty clutching the blanket.

Friends and spectators were already urging exhausted rafters toward the celebrations. Doris, my clinic assistant and good conscience, rushed up to us all smiles. She threw her arms around my middle in an uncharacteristic bear hug before smothering her daughter, Barb, with a proud-mama kiss. More well-wishers descended to offer congratulations—even shaking from the frigid cold, I felt a warmth knowing that in just a couple of years I'd accumulated so many dear friends.

Marcie stayed close by me, happy to bask in the attention, too, though most of these people were strangers to her. A summer student from veterinary college in Saskatoon, she had been working for the federal veterinary inspector in Creston and spending every spare moment with me viewing cases at my clinic. She had only been in the Kootenays for four weeks, but I was hoping she'd consider coming back after her graduation. And by the look on her rose-cheeked face, I had reason to have high hopes.

I looked around for Cory, finally spotting him over the heads of the crowd (one of the perks of my near seven-foot stature). My friend was tailing the migrating mob, a blanket draped over his slumped shoulders.

"Cory!" I called out. I wanted him to enjoy the rewards of our success as much as Marcie, Barb, and I were.

He turned and waved with a smile, just to say, *I'm fine*. We knew each other well enough to reduce a conversation to this sign language. He had been one of my best friends through four years in veterinary college. Together, we had slogged through countless hours of hitting the books, and a fair number of late nights downing beer. Cory was the kind of unassuming friend I imagined everyone deserved. He was someone for whom school wasn't easy—not that socializing was all that easy for him, either. So he tended to go with the flow, work when he really needed to, and simply be an all-around nice guy. I guess Cory was happy to take a back seat on the ride of life. At least that's how it seemed to me at the time.

"Beer! Horny Owl! Now!" The voice was unmistakeable. George Huscroft, the irascible redheaded lumberjack, was again determined to lead the charge. We had just finished downing some of Dick Sommerfeld's barbecued beef and were starting to warm up.

George had seemingly made a total recovery from a close call

14

at Keeney's Hole when his raft was swept beneath a logjam. Before I got to him, he had been clinging to a huge snag to keep from going under. He must have been somewhat disappointed at his failure to finish the race—after all, he had been determined that this was going to be the year for him to claim first prize. Although he had taunted me relentlessly about this race being "no place for a woman," he had grudgingly admitted, "Marcie did pretty good out there today."

He was right—she had done pretty good out there. We all had. But none of us was feeling much like beer right now.

"Ya don't want to be party-poopers," cautioned George. "Just a quick one for the road."

No…we certainly wouldn't want to be party-poopers.

Vehicles were parked on both sides of the street for the entire length of the block on the far side of the railway tracks. A constant flow of people indicated we had found the right place. A sign in big red letters on the squat white building read simply *HOTEL*. In smaller painted letters, over the little door at the left, was scrawled *Horny Owl Saloon*.

A train whistle blared; a diesel engine revved only fifty yards away. There was a clang, clang, clang as boxcars were coupled in the sorting yard. Everyone in my Volkswagen looked as tired as I felt. No one lifted a finger. The door to the Horny Owl was open, and even from across the street, I could see the room was packed.

"Come on. Let's do this," I urged my reluctant partners.

Any other day, the proprietor would be lucky to see half a dozen people in his establishment. Today, we'd be lucky to find a seat. I willed my shaky legs up the five steps to the door—my knees were still not fond of bending.

The tiny bar was bulging at the seams. People yelled in each other's ears to be heard above the blaring country music. The air was heavy with cigarette smoke and the smell of spilled beer. We stood at the doorway for a moment surveying the crowd, almost hoping we wouldn't find our crew so we could head home and collapse.

"Hey, Doc!" It was the redheaded dynamo. Leaning against a long table in the centre of the room, he waved his white cowboy hat at us. "We got a few chairs here!"

The four of us squeezed in with the Lougheeds (Dave had finished third in the race) and George and his wife, Linda. I sat down against one of the heavy timber pillars on which was nailed an old crosscut saw and half a dozen leghold traps.

"George has been defending these chairs against all comers!" shouted Dave Lougheed. "Glad you finally got here. Thought we were in for a brawl over 'em a few minutes ago." He glanced at the table next to him—a crew of lumberjacks as rough in appearance as George, but not half as friendly. "These guys over here are looking for trouble, and George seems a bit feisty after his dip in the river."

George shot Lougheed a look but refused to give him the satisfaction of a response.

"Have a beer, you guys!" George grabbed a pitcher and filled a glass for each of us. "Sure glad ya came along when ya did this afternoon, Doc." He was slurring his words noticeably. "Not sure how much longer I coulda held on to that log."

I sipped my brew, willing it to turn into a hot rum toddy. I gazed around the saloon wondering about the wild times it had witnessed since the turn of the century. Now, it saw only a fraction of its former splendour on this one day a year. I squinted in the dim light. The walls were covered in dark wood panelling. Old lanterns hung from overhead beams. Stuffed creatures were everywhere—ducks and hawks perched side by side over a huge stone fireplace; a four-point buck stared vacantly from its place in the corner. One wall was plastered with old license plates, and a sign proclaimed: *No Clock, No Phone, No Address—Retired!*

"How are you doing, Marcie? You warming up yet?" I rested my hand on her arm; she was still shivering. She smiled and

16

nodded. She had hardly said a word since we were thrown into the drink. I wondered what she was thinking—was she being aloof because I was obviously attracted to her? She was a good-looking woman, and we had a lot in common, but...

George got up and staggered across the bar toward the can. Good idea—this beer was travelling right through me. I followed in his wake, several steps behind. He disappeared through the men's room door before I entered to find the long lineup for the wooden stall and urinals. A pithy verse stencilled on the wall caught my attention: *Little drops of water on the toilet floor / Ruin the linoleum and make the barmaid sore / So all you kind gentlemen / Before the water flows / Measure the distance according to your hose.*

I saw the back of George's distinctive white hat, still plunked squarely on his head. He'd somehow managed to bypass the queue and was standing at a urinal next to one of the loggers that Lougheed had pointed out, a burly man in a black leather jacket. That was George—a guy who could charm a raging grizzly...or if charm didn't work, he'd try his best to kick its butt.

"So you're loggin' up the Goat, are ya?" George said. "Hear you been running your own crew."

The man in black didn't answer, and George didn't seem to notice as he continued on in a booming voice. "Yeah, I'm fallin' for Mel Faurot right now. Pretty good work. Good guy. Just do your thing, you get paid." Still no comment. "Hey, if you ever need a good faller, I like workin' in that country."

"Sorry," came the reply in a heavy French accent, "I only hire da real man."

George's shoulders straightened. My heart sank—this would not end well. Without giving George even a glance, the man in black zipped up and exited. By the time George turned to face me, his face was flushed. But he smiled, as though nothing was wrong at all.

"See you back at the table, Dave."

I nodded. George left calmly. There was gonna be a gunfight.

The atmosphere had changed considerably by the time I returned to my seat. Everyone around the table looked uncomfortable, and George had a sullen expression on his face.

"Just settle down, big fella. Gagnon's not worth it," Lougheed muttered to his friend. "Just thinks he's a big shot 'cause he has his own crew. Plus, he's been drinking."

"Uh huh." That was all George said in return before he stood and strode to the bar, empty pitcher in hand.

"Look out." Lougheed leaned close to my ear. "I've been around this big redheaded bugger for a lot of years, and when he gets that look in his eyes, it's not good."

"Maybe it's time to leave," Marcie suggested.

"Maybe," Cory agreed.

We were getting up from the table when George returned. "Drink up, Doc! Ya bailed me out big time today. Least ya can do is let me buy ya a beer."

I knew he wouldn't take no for an answer. I glanced at Marcie and polished off what remained in my glass. George filled it to the brim. Marcie and Cory were already standing. She gave me a look that said *Let's go*. But she didn't know George Huscroft like I knew George Huscroft.

Things were getting rowdier by the minute. The adjacent table, where George's French-speaking compatriot sat, was the loudest. Next to him sat a lithe fellow in his late twenties, who looked at us and made some comment I couldn't catch. He then clapped Gagnon on the back and hooted with laughter.

The man in black didn't laugh at the joke and seemed to appreciate the slap on the back even less. When the younger man stood up momentarily with his beer, Gagnon pulled the chair out from under him. He hit the floor ass-first, sending the contents of his glass through the air to douse everyone at our table. George's wife jumped up with beer dripping from the end of her nose. George, who was still making the rounds with his pitcher, resolutely set it down. Wiping beer from his bushy beard and the front of his fancy white shirt, he carefully hung his hat on the set of antlers over his head.

"Outside, Gagnon!" he roared. He may not have won the race today, but he had no intention of losing this fight.

The burly man grinned at his drinking buddies and followed George to the exit. They had no sooner reached the door than Gagnon swung at George. George ducked aside, surprisingly agile given his size and inebriated state. In turn, he smoked the guy. Gagnon fell like a tree, landing hard on the floor flat on his back. George went to pounce on him, but Gagnon saw him coming and lifted his leg. His boot caught George in the chest, sending the unsuspecting redhead backwards out the open door and down the front stairs.

We reached the steps in time to see Gagnon land a haymaker over George's left eye. George dropped to his knees. Dazed, and bleeding from the road rash on the side of his face, the cowboy stared at his opponent for what seemed an eternity. Then something snapped in him, and he began thumping on Gagnon. The logging boss fell over backwards; George jumped on him like a crazed pit bull.

The crowd poured out of the bar, and from that moment on, things got really out of hand. A husky young man—one of Gagnon's crew—threw down his hamburger and fired a kick at George's head. George crumpled and covered his head as the guy continued to pummel him. I grabbed the obnoxious kid by his shirt and hurled him across the yard. He crashed into a car and landed in a heap. Enraged, he got up slowly, ready for a fight. Lifting his dukes, he took a step in my direction.

"Are you really sure that's what you want to do?" I was surprised by the tone of Marcie's voice. She was standing at the top of the stairs directing her advice to the young ruffian. "You look smarter than that."

The man stopped short. Gagnon struggled to his feet and aimed a kick at George as he lay on his side on the ground.

19

"Enough of that!" shouted Lougheed. Jumping down the steps, he whirled the logger around and nailed him squarely on the jaw. Gagnon sank to his knees. No one else moved.

Things settled down quickly after the scuffle. The bar patrons huddled in groups, mumbling in hushed tones. Linda was dabbing at George's bruised face with napkins from the bar. His left eye was swollen shut. Blood oozed from raw areas on his forehead and cheek and trickled down his beard. His good eye watered as he wobbled back and forth trying to focus on me.

"Did ya see that, Doc?" He shook his fist for effect. "I took his best punch."

"You've had a hell of a day, George."

"Uh huh," George agreed. "And aren't you gonna say nothin', Marcie?"

Marcie's eyes widened, unclear what he was getting at.

"You know, you should just say it. Here I tell you the race is no place for a woman—then you finish it and I don't. I have to get my sorry ass rescued, only to land on it again in a bar fight. So go ahead…rub my nose in it good."

"Oh." Marcie looked at me, then back at George. "Well, I think if you could see your nose right now, you'd agree…you've had your nose rubbed in it enough today."

It was true…His nose was a bruised and bloody mess. George laughed so hard that Linda had to step back from her nursing duties.

"She's a keeper, Dave! She's a keeper!" he bellowed.

I smiled at Marcie. I was beginning to see just how right George was about her. Marcie was a keeper.

Bacillus at Hurfords

"How could a case of mastitis possibly get so far ahead of them?" asked Marcie.

"That's a good question." We had just left Isolum Farms, and the sight of 113's udder was firmly imprinted on my mind. "I can only think of two possibilities: one, that we're dealing with a real super bug; the other, that the boys were asleep at the switch, not really paying attention when they ran her through this morning."

The look on her face was one of revulsion. "I've never seen anything like this before. That udder was so cold, so hard—like a block of wood."

"If it makes you feel any better, she's the worst case I've seen. I'm not sure how an udder could look more disgusting. I don't think she has a hope in hell of making it."

"What about the fluids and chloramphenicol?"

"Never say never, but she's in pretty rough shape. When I hit the vein to start the IV, the fluid that came from her looked more like port wine than blood. Unless I miss my guess, she'll be my first call of the morning. Herb has me do a post-mortem on everything that dies on the place."

Marcie stared absently out the car window at a flock of geese that circled for a landing over the drainage ditch parallelling the gravel road.

"What organism would you expect to cause a mastitis that severe?"

I was pushing my summer helper to dredge up particulars from her third-year medicine course. I could just picture Otto

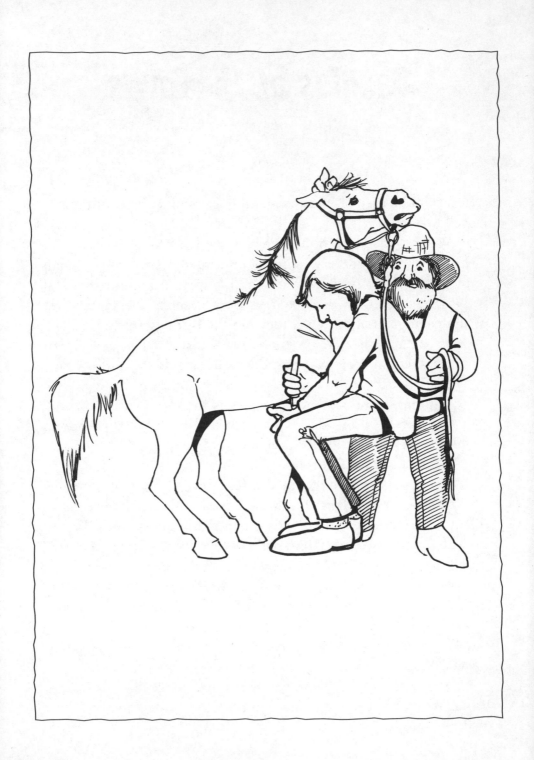

Radostits, the instructor we had both trained under, standing at the front of the lecture theatre fishing for differential diagnoses. Back at the vet college, the names of all those bacteria seemed so theoretical. Now that one of my best friends was in a fight to save another cow and maybe his livelihood, the academics suddenly took on more meaning.

We had left Dan Hurford to maintain a five-gallon intravenous drip on an animal that was struggling to stay alive. Manure poured from the cow's rectum like water, and her eyes were sunken so deeply into her head that one would have sworn she'd been starving for weeks. This was the second case we had fought with in less than a month.

"Would a staph look like that?" Marcie's tone was hesitant.

"It certainly has to be on the list of differentials…I've seen a few acute cases that produced a watery mastitis like this one, but none that caused gangrene."

I braked at the end of the long driveway to Tsolum Farms. A grain truck was heading north toward town. I waved to Ken Hanson as he barrelled by in the huge blue tandem, then swung onto Reclamation Road to follow him "What else?"

"E. coli and klebsiella?" Marcie looked uncomfortable—she didn't like it much when I quizzed her this way.

"You bet! I'd put my money on E. coli. I've never seen one cause that much tissue death before, though. Man, was it gross."

"I know…and there was that terrible odour about her." Marcie wrinkled her nose. "She smelled like she'd already been dead for a few days."

We drove past the old ferry landing and turned west toward the new bypass road that had replaced it.

"One would have to keep in mind some of the anaerobes, too," I muttered as an afterthought. "Even though there was no gas in the quarter, I don't think we can totally rule out some sort of clostridia."

I drove on in silence, wracking my brain for a diagnosis.

Pondering each organism for a few moments, I could think of an argument to discard each one of them. The only time I had ever seen an udder quite like the one on this cow was the one I had done a post-mortem on the week before. I would have sworn the dark line of tissue death expanded into new territory as we watched. What a horrible feeling, knowing that even though it was still attached to the critter's body, the majority of the udder was already dead.

I twigged to a conversation that I had had with John Hopkins at last fall's B.C. veterinary convention. He and Trevor Clarkson had talked about cases of gangrenous mastitis that they had just dealt with. Both seasoned dairy practitioners from the Fraser Valley, they were part of a small group of veterinarians who had tried to make me feel at home in their conversation. I remembered the feeling of revulsion I had when Trevor told us about taking a pair of scissors and cutting a cow's teat off flush to her udder. Allowing for drainage of the toxins from the udder made sense, but never would I have considered it myself...until today.

I could still see the look on Marcie's face when I had returned from the car with a pair of scissors and whacked off 113's two rear teats. After becoming accustomed to seeing blood run in a steady stream from even a tiny cut on a teat, it was amazing to me that not a drop appeared on the blue-black margin of the wound. The only discharge was the foul-smelling maroon-coloured fluid that oozed from the teat cistern itself.

I warned Dan that he'd have to dig the straw right down to the concrete and lime the pen immediately to prevent the spread of this terrible bug. I was sure the fact that Marcie and I had scrubbed our boots for five minutes after finishing with the cow had impressed on Dan the gravity of the situation. I couldn't suppress the overwhelming feeling that this pathogen was something out of the ordinary and deserved special respect.

I noticed that the skin on my hands was still wrinkled and waterlogged from scrubbing. At times like this, I knew I shouldn't touch a sick critter without rubber gloves. I wasn't aware of any more dairy calls today—there was no way I wanted to be a source of contamination for my other clients! Our coveralls would have to be soaked for hours in disinfectant before being washed.

It was a few minutes after five when we arrived back at the office. Doris glanced longingly at her watch. "It looks like I'm going to get out of here on time tonight."

During the three years she had been my nurse, receptionist, and office manager, she had never been a clock-watcher—except on Tuesdays. This week saw the beginning of the women's league roll-off at the bowling alley, and Doris was determined that she and the girls were going all the way this year.

"Bill Hook wants you to give him a ring at the Canyon Store. His son's horse is lame, and he wants to talk to you about it."

I rang the store as Doris dashed out the door. A man answered.

"Hi, Bill. This is Dave Perrin returning your call."

"Hello, Dave. Thanks for getting back to me. Billy's mare seems to have injured herself. Last Saturday he went for a bit of a ride and came back after a few minutes because Petronella limped the whole time. I told him to give her some rest and see if she didn't improve. He just came in an hour ago really upset. The horse won't even touch her foot to the ground."

"Did it happen gradually, or did she suddenly take a turn for the worse?"

"To be honest with you, I can't answer that. We took off for a few days to the lake and only just got back this afternoon. Billy's fit to be tied. I went out there to check the horse myself a few minutes ago. It looks bad to me…She just holds the foot up in the air and waves it around."

"I can come have a look right now if you like. It sounds as if she should have attention as soon as possible."

"I'd appreciate that. I'll call a friend to meet you and give you a hand…I'll have to stay here and man the store. Petronella will be in Ray Roper's pasture, if you know where that is."

"I do. I have a sample to get off to the lab, but I should make it to Canyon in about forty-five minutes."

"Great! Hope it's nothing serious. Billy thinks the world of that horse. We got her from Eleanor Blair…as you can tell, she named her."

I chuckled. Nell had such unique names for her critters. "I'll stop at the store when we're done and let you know what I found."

It was almost six by the time I got the Tsolum samples on the bus to the lab, and Marcie and I were off to Canyon. As we passed Eleanor's yard, I could see that she had Honey saddled and hard at work. A young girl decked out in a bowler hat and English riding habit posted in a circle under my friend's watchful eye. I waved and glanced in the rear-view mirror. I noticed Eleanor scurry to the fence and crane her neck as she followed my progress down her neighbour's lane. I knew it would drive her mad trying to figure out what I was doing next door.

A black horse I presumed to be Petronella was standing in the corner of the pasture. Lounging next to her was a husky man with a bushy red beard. I smiled at the silhouette beneath the huge cowboy hat and looked across at Marcie.

"It's your old buddy, George."

Marcie smiled half-heartedly and got out of the car.

"Hi there, cowboy. You sure look in better shape than the last time we saw you!"

He smiled. The very thought of the Yahk bar episode made his pale blue eyes sparkle. "Hi there, Dave…Hi, Marcie. Yeah, I wasn't lookin' too good by the time you guys left, but that was nothin'—you shoulda seen me the next day. My eyes were swoll shut and my face was a mess of scabs. It took all month ta get back ta normal. It was lucky I was out in camp."

I had been observing the mare as we approached. Ears back, she was staring straight ahead with a look of dejection. She bore her full weight on her left front foot, resting the heel of her right front loosely on the ground. I stroked her neck a few times, then reached down to rest my hand on the top of her forward foot. She immediately picked it up and waved it erratically back and forth.

"Easy, girl...easy," I said quietly, as the animal struggled to keep me from getting hold of her limb. I abandoned the sore foot for a moment.

"Settle down, Petronella!" George gave the unhappy horse a no-nonsense look and took firm command of the halter. "Poor critter. Who the hell would give a horse a name like that?"

"Is there any increase in heat?" Marcie asked, watching the proceedings intently and trying her best to ignore George.

"Not that I can detect." I grasped the foot firmly and prodded along the margin of the hoof with the tip of my thumb looking for evidence of pain or swelling. When I found nothing unusual, I flexed the foot, flipped the hoof over, and pulled it tight to my body. I probed the heel and the leathery structure called the frog, searching for signs of moisture or discoloration. I squeezed across the back of the horse's heel, and she whipped the foot from my hand.

"Easy there, Petronella," George chimed. "She sure is sore. Do you think she broke something?"

"Not impossible." I turned to Marcie. "Can you hand me the hoof knife?"

She pulled a pair of knives from her back pocket and handed me one. I scraped the surface of the sole, looking for anything out of the ordinary. The horse ripped and pulled constantly at her foot in an attempt to free herself. When I persisted, she settled somewhat and I continued to scrape. I glanced up from my crouched position to see that George had the horse's ear securely in his grasp. He was giving old Petronella something else to focus her attention on. "See anything?" he asked.

I had the bottom of the foot completely pared down to a solid white texture, had cleaned out the sulcus where the leathery frog met the horn of the sole, and still found nothing.

"Pass me the hoof tester, Marcie, please."

She handed me the unwieldy-looking pincers. I spread the huge jaws open and positioned them in such a manner that one tip contacted the top of the hoof wall and the other applied pressure to the sole. Gingerly putting tension on the handles, I worked my way in a circular fashion around the perimeter. Each time I increased the pressure, the horse flinched and gave a slight tug on the leg.

"By God, those are sure wicked-lookin' things." George instinctively tightened his grip on Petronella's halter.

I routinely squeezed away at the entire sole surface, taking note of the horse's reaction to each compression. Whenever I applied even the slightest pressure to an area a few inches in front of the frog, she struggled vehemently. I scraped at the area with the hoof knife, trying to convince myself that it was slightly discoloured. I applied the hoof tester one more time. Petronella reared back and pulled herself off the ground, dragging the determined redhead along with her.

"Yer sure doin' somethin' she doesn't like." A bead of sweat ran down George's forehead as he manhandled the horse back to the ground. Pushing his cowboy hat to the back of his head, he adjusted his right hand on the horse's halter for a better purchase and resumed his grasp of the ear with the left.

"It appears so," I grunted, wrestling the foot firmly to my leg. Timing my strokes with the knife to the animal's constant jerking, I carved a circular pattern in the sole over the most sensitive area. Several times Petronella exploded in a fit of temper. Each time we rode out her protest and returned to the persistent erosion of the sole surface.

"You diggin' to China?" George looked askance at the circular depression that was now taking on a pinkish hue.

"Not quite." I stubbornly held onto Petronella's foot as she reared again, then bent down for a closer look at the area I was abusing. "Have a look at this." I motioned for Marcie to lean closer, then moved back so George could get a better view. "See how the centre is starting to look a bit darker—how it's almost brown rather than pink?"

"Yeah. What does that mean?" George watched attentively.

"I hope it means we have an abscess under here."

I pressed on the thin layer of sole with my index finger, and Petronella reacted as if I had jabbed her with a needle. I poised my knife over the discoloration, and with a quick flick of my wrist, carved the centre from it. A jet of pus shot from the wound, and the mare struggled to gain her freedom.

"Easy, girl. It's all over now…it's all over. That should feel better with all that pressure gone."

The horse waved her foot in the air as pus and blood dripped from the tip of her toe. I stroked her neck as she calmed down and rested her sore foot on the ground. My hand came away moist—she had worked up a sweat.

"Let's keep her from stepping on it too much until I get it bandaged."

"How in the devil did you know that was there, Dave?" The cowboy's tone was one of awe. "I couldn't see a thing where you were diggin'."

"I had to talk myself into it, George. Had a gut feeling—and Petronella kept telling me I was right."

I packed the wound with ointment and covered it with gauze before swaddling the foot with an adhesive bandage. Almost immediately, the horse straightened her right front leg and began to bear weight.

The Hooks were ecstatic to hear that Petronella's condition would only be a temporary setback. I dropped Marcie off at her landlady's home in Erickson and headed to the office.

What a gorgeous evening. As I drove through the orchard properties, I tried convincing myself to pick up my faithful friend Lug from the apartment and head out to my farm. But no matter how hard I tried, I just couldn't get the sight of 113's rotting udder from my mind. Never had I seen anything similar to this type of mastitis. I thought the first case was some sort of aberration, but here was another one.

I parked in the lot and headed right to the back room of the clinic. Lug met me at the front door and circled excitedly around me as I made my way across the office. I mechanically roughed his ears, then began thumbing through the lab reports on the clip-board. I stopped when I got to the one on Tsolum Farms. I read through the findings of the post-mortem report on cow #93—about the severe degenerative changes and the tissue death.

I read the culture report again. My eyes kept coming back to focus on the mention of the organism, *Bacillus cereus*. It was a bug I had never heard of before reading this report. The dissertation went on to suggest that the bacteria was not commonly known as a cause of mastitis and must obviously have been a contaminant in the sample.

I thought back to the cow. Number 93 had been an older animal, but Herb swore up and down that she had never had a previous problem with mastitis. The farm records indicated she had been treated with antibiotics on drying off, but that was part of a dry-cow therapy program that I had introduced. Infusing cows as they completed their last lactation was a means of catching chronic or subclinical cases of mastitis that insidiously cut into a cow's production.

The Hurford boys claimed that they had taken enough from her at first milking to ease tension on the udder. They had intentionally not stripped her for fear of inducing milk fever. No one had seen anything unusual at the time. At the following milking, all quarters were hard and obviously painful. When David tried milking her, he found only red watery fluid. He was surprised that the hindquarters felt as cold as ice. The cow was shaky on her feet and was discharging a watery diarrhea.

By the time I got there two hours later, #93 was moribund. Her temperature was a degree below normal and stool poured from her rectum like water. I remembered feeling at the time that it was the worst case of coliform mastitis that I had ever seen. I started antibiotic therapy. When I left, intravenous fluids were pouring into her vein. She was dead inside of two hours.

I could see her corpse stretched out waiting for me at the edge of the cornfield. Her udder had been as hard as a rock, but the overlying skin was not as affected to the same degree as #113's was now.

I remembered my first reading of the lab report—how my ears had burned at the suggestion of a contaminant. I read the report over and over, hoping that something I had missed would jump from the paper and solve my dilemma.

I pulled my copy of *Veterinary Medicine* by Blood and Henderson from the shelf. I opened the well-worn text to the index and the subtitle "Gangrenous Mastitis." Nothing on *Bacillus cereus*…nothing that made me the least bit wiser.

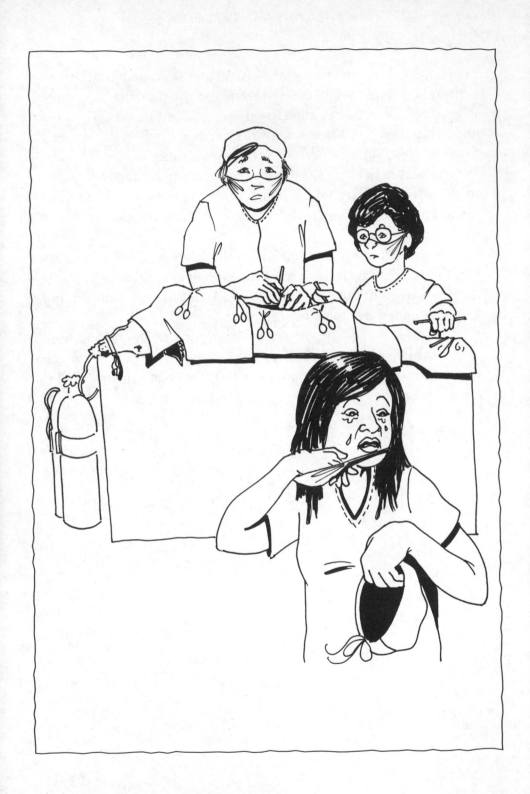

Gut Feeling

"Trixie's just not herself, Dr. Perrin. If you could have seen her only a few months ago, you'd understand how much she's failed. She's always been such an active dog, but the last while she's done nothing but lie around."

I studied my new patient. The collie-cross bitch certainly didn't look like an animal that hadn't eaten in weeks. Sitting bolt upright, she focused worried eyes on her owner and diligently avoided the temptation of looking in my direction. She trembled. Whether she was feeling up to par or not, the dog was sharp enough to know she was at the doctor's office.

"Trixie's the smartest dog we've ever had," Sonja Wittmoser affirmed.

She addressed her husband who was standing just inside the door. "Isn't that right, Siggy?...We'll be sitting at home and she'll come up and let me know she wants something. All I have to do is ask her what she needs and she tells me. Watch this—I'll ask her if she's hungry..."

The woman held her fingers over the dog's nose by way of demonstration. "If she's hungry, she wiggles her bum back and forth and barks at me." Sonja continued addressing her pet in a most enthusiastic fashion. "Do you want a piece of apple? A carrot? A doggie biscuit?"

Returning her attention to me, she said, "The moment I hit on what she wants, she wags her tail and gives me a little woof."

The dog shot her mistress a look of disinterest and plunked with a sigh on the waiting room floor. "See that—that's not our

Trixie. Siggy and I are sure there's something seriously amiss...We've asked around in Crawford Bay—we're building a new home there—and everyone tells us to bring her to you. We want to know what's wrong with her."

Sonja studied my face as if it were part of her preliminary evaluation. Here was a person used to getting her own way. She sank to the carpet and took the dog's head in her hands.

"What's wrong with you, Trixie? Won't you tell Momma?"

There was certainly no doubting this woman's loving concern for her pet. Although she looked as if she'd just rushed over from a session at the beauty parlour, here she was kneeling on a floor that had seen several canine clients already this day. She gently stroked the animal's head, not the least bit concerned about the layer of dog hair that was accumulating on her checkered wool skirt.

I was about to question Mrs. Wittmoser further about Trixie's medical history when the door crashed open. In stumbled my father's cousin. They shared the same name—Marshall—a handle that had apparently been passed down for generations in Grandma's Cameron lineage. Marsh appeared to be on the losing end of a long bender—his clothes were rumpled and his face was covered with several days' growth of stubble. He stepped around Mr. Wittmoser and gravitated to the corner. Leaning against the wall for support, he slowly settled to the waiting room bench.

When Marsh realized that he was the focus of attention, he flushed and glanced apprehensively toward the office.

"The girls in, Dave?" he muttered.

"Sorry, Marsh...Doris and Shirley are gone for the day. The office is actually closed...I'm just here on an emergency."

He blinked several times as if having difficulty processing the information. "Do you think I could have my fiver?"

Marsh was referring to the five-dollar bill that we usually had hidden away in the cash drawer. It had simply become the floating five—the five dollars he borrowed for a taxi ride home at the end of a toot. Only if he had returned it after the last transaction could he expect it to be there waiting for him.

"So you're out of the camp now?"

It had been six months since I'd seen him here in this shape. Prone to binge drinking, Marsh went through long dry spells where he abandoned the bottle and returned to his job as a camp cook.

"Yeah, finished up last week." He yawned, closed his eyes reflexively, and moaned.

I flushed as the scent of stale booze washed over us like a wave. I turned to Sonja. "I'll just be a second, if you don't mind."

She smiled. "Go right ahead."

I picked up the phone and rang Creston Taxi. Bill was at home and he promised to come right over. I plucked the five-dollar bill from the little white file box where Doris and Shirley kept it and returned to Marsh.

He sat there quietly with his eyes focused on Trixie. As I approached, he addressed Mrs. Wittmoser. "Had a dog just like yours once, lady." He smiled. "She was a good one."

"Here you go, Marsh." I handed him the five note.

"Thanks, Dave…I'll bring it back tomorrow."

He got up and took a few unsteady steps toward the door.

"I called the taxi…You be here when it arrives."

"Couldn't I wait across the street?"

I knew that nothing would suit him better than to wait for the taxi in John Shean's bar.

"You know the deal, Marsh. I pay for the taxi home…Bill will be here in a minute."

He nodded sadly. I watched him shuffle onto the street. What a waste—Marsh was one of the nicest men you could ever want to meet. Drunk or sober, he'd give you the shirt off his back. When he was off the bottle, he worked like a hound to try and get back on top, and not once had he failed to return the money that he borrowed.

I contemplated Mrs. Wittmoser's ring-laden fingers as she picked at a knot of hair under Trixie's chin.

"You say that she's been examined by other veterinarians? Do you have any record of the workup that was done?"

"I have her records here." The tall, sturdily built man watching from the doorway extended a manila envelope. I opened the packet and thumbed through the photocopied material. His eyes shifted constantly from the dog to me and back to the dog again.

"I'm Siggy," he said presenting his hand. It was the first time he had actually offered input. "As you can see, we took her to several different clinics. No one seems to be able to put their finger on what's going on. Our regular vet just didn't seem concerned enough, so we took her elsewhere. Sonja and I know our dog…We're convinced that there's something wrong."

"I see that there was a series of X-rays done—"

"Yes, they were taken this Thursday." Mr. Wittmoser's face was drawn. "I was convinced they were going to show us what was happening. Trixie actually ate a few pieces of carrot and some dog food that morning, but she vomited it right after. That was the final straw for me. I took the day off work just to try and get to the bottom of it, but the doctor didn't come up with anything conclusive…She mentioned something about a lot of gas—that if Trixie didn't improve, we should consider a barium series."

Kneeling beside the dog, I gently pinched the skin on her brow. It remained tented. I took a peek into her eyes, then rolled up her lip to press on her gums.

"What are you looking for?" Sonja was obviously the type of client who wanted a blow-by-blow description of my administrations.

"She looks a bit anemic…and she's definitely dehydrated."

"That's not surprising." Siggy shook his head slowly from side to side. "She hasn't had a thing to drink since last night. I held a dish of water up to her nose…Even then, it was as if she took a lap just to please me."

Seeming weary, the man suddenly sank to the waiting room bench. "I'm an architect and I still run a business in Calgary. We're back and forth a lot right now. Usually when we're making the trip down to the Kootenays, Trixie sits quietly until we get through Cranbrook. But we just can't get by Moyie Lake without her creating such a fuss that we have to let her out for a run. She always has her radar turned on…Today she never even noticed till we got to Creston and stopped here."

"So she's gone downhill significantly in the last few days?" I ran my hands up and down the dog's body, petting her and gently prodding in search of enlarged lymph nodes or lumps that didn't belong.

"At first there were just moments when she didn't seem herself," Sonja interjected. "These last three or four days, she hasn't had many good ones."

"You mentioned that she vomited the other day. How often has she thrown up…How long has it been since she really ate as if she were hungry?"

"When was it that I first asked you if she was losing weight, hon? I'd say about two weeks, wouldn't you?"

Siggy scratched his head thoughtfully. "It's been all of that. Can you give me that blue form, Doctor? That's the one from our regular vet. We were there in the middle of April for a checkup and he couldn't find anything. I know I'd been concerned about her for a few days already—she just wasn't eating as well as she should have been."

I went back through the records. "What can you tell me about this episode at the end of March?" I passed the page to Siggy. "It says she was hit by a car. Did you see it happen?"

"I did…I was walking her that night. We were almost to the park and I took her lead off. She was so excited about getting out there for her run that she darted out in front of a little Toyota just when it was leaving the parking lot. It didn't amount to much. She hit the bumper, and it sort of threw her to the side. The lady stopped right away. It scared all of us. Our vet checked Trixie over and couldn't find anything. It never slowed her down in the least. In fact, she was so rambunctious when I took her to the clinic that I felt kind of silly for even bothering them."

I gently palpated Trixie's abdomen. For a dog that hadn't eaten in days, her tummy felt full. I pressed in with my fingers first on one side, then the other. Finally I tried touching the indentation of my fingers on the opposite side. There was always something in the way—loop after loop of gas-filled bowel.

"She doesn't like that," Sonja observed with a look of concern. "Did you find something?"

"I'm not sure, but I noticed on the last checkup in Calgary the vet mentions discomfort on deep palpation."

"That's why she did the X-rays," Siggy interjected.

"There's more gas than I'd expect for a dog that hasn't eaten for a week, and she definitely doesn't like this."

I directed my fingertips forward, searching for a lump that could represent a foreign body. The dog squirmed uncomfortably and glared at me in protest. "There has to be something, the way she's acting."

"What do you suggest, Doctor?" It was obvious that Sonja was determined to get an immediate resolution to Trixie's problem.

"We need to get her started on intravenous fluids to get her rehydrated. My gut feeling is that we're dealing with some sort of blockage. She's definitely uncomfortable when I palpate her bowels, and that amount of gas is certainly not normal."

"Are you suggesting surgery?" Siggy asked.

"The way I see it, we have two alternatives." I stood up and leaned against the counter. "We can either do a barium series to search for a blockage, or we can proceed with an exploratory. This has apparently been going on for some time and doesn't appear to be something simple. If it were, I'm sure one of the other veterinarians would have put a finger on the problem. If we do find a blockage, we'll still have to do something about it."

Siggy stared thoughtfully at Trixie and stooped to pet her. "I just don't understand why if there was something wrong, it didn't show up on the X-ray."

"Sometimes plastic or something like a cone from an evergreen won't show up well in a radiograph. It's also possible that something happened to cause a displacement when she got bumped by that car."

The couple looked apprehensively at one another.

"Let's get her on the exam table so I can start an intravenous. No matter what we do, she needs fluids."

I gathered together what I needed for the intravenous set-up while the Wittmosers coaxed poor Trixie further into enemy territory.

"Come on, sweetie." Sonja knelt on the examination room floor enthusiastically slapping her thighs with her hands. "Come see Momma. There's a girl…there's a girl."

Creeping hesitantly toward her mistress, the dog eyed me uneasily. She had obviously garnered little love for veterinarians through her recent associations with them.

By the time I had returned with the IV stand and had the administration set ready to go, Siggy had wrestled the reluctant dog onto the table. The man seemed distressed—as if he wanted to just grab his beloved pet and make a run for it.

I started the clippers and bared a small portion of Trixie's fore arm. Siggy blanched. He took a step back as I ran an alcohol swab back and forth over the area. I removed the catheter from its sterile packaging and grasped the plastic shield in my teeth. The moment I exposed the shaft of the catheter, the man was gone.

"Siggy's not too big on this sort of thing," Sonja observed dryly. "How would you like me to hold her?" She stepped forward and held her pet's head as I plunged the needle into the vein.

"We've decided that we'd like to go ahead with an exploratory."

The couple had just returned from lunch. Sonja walked into

the surgery and knelt in front of the kennel where Trixie lay stretched out on her side. Siggy stood near the doorway, gazing apprehensively at the intravenous apparatus that slowly dripped away.

"We need some sort of resolution, one way or the other," Sonja said with determination. "We just can't watch her waste away in front of our eyes."

"I'll call my assistant and see if she can come back to help us."

It was three-thirty. Poor Doris had left for home a few minutes after noon for her weekend break, but I knew she wouldn't hesitate if I asked her to return.

I medicated Trixie. She lay stretched out on her side in the surgery kennel, fast asleep. Doris breezed in and soon had the drapes and surgery packs sitting in readiness on the counter.

"You can stay and watch if you wish," I said to Sonja. "We may need to get some direction once we're in there."

"I'd like that," she said and waved to Siggy.

"I'll go down to the builders' supply and line up some of the materials we need for the deck," he called with relief as he headed out the door.

I woke the dog from her drug-induced slumber and lifted her onto the table. Slipping the mask over her muzzle, I stroked her head as she temporarily objected to inhaling the sweet-smelling combination of gases. Within five minutes she was sound asleep. I introduced a tube down her trachea, hooked her up to the anesthetic machine, and adjusted the levels of nitrous oxide, halothane, and oxygen. Doris clipped the hair from her abdomen and Sonja gathered it with the vacuum. Aside from her obvious irritation with the cap and mask that we insisted upon, Sonja seemed calm and collected as we proceeded with the preparation.

By the time Doris had finished the final scrub of the dog, I had finished mine, and she helped me slip into my gown and gloves. I felt comfortable with Sonja viewing the surgery. Although she was very fond of her pet, she seemed to be able to detach herself enough to stand back and observe unobtrusively.

I positioned a drape at Trixie's pubis and another at her sternum to give me as much exposure as possible. Placing the side drapes, I grasped the corner clamps to apply them. Sonja flinched as each clamp clicked and the pincers drove through her dog's skin.

I covered the remainder of the table with a large throw drape, prepared the tray, and laid out the instruments. I locked a blade into a scalpel handle and incised from Trixie's umbilicus to her pelvis. The moment I cut through the peritoneum, I knew I was in trouble.

The bowel, which normally could be followed from the duodenum as it left the stomach to the colon where it joined the rectum, was one solid lump.

"Oh no."

I stared in horror at the mass of adhesions. How could a dog that outwardly seemed normal have things so badly screwed up?

Sonja scratched uncomfortably at her mask. "What's going on? That's not good, is it?"

I lengthened the incision and struggled to lift the tangled conglomerate of bowels at least partway out of the abdomen.

"No way." I glanced uneasily from Doris to Sonja. "This doesn't look good."

I worked my fingers between what I thought to be sections of jejunum— part of the small intestine between the duodenum and ileum—and struggled to separate them. Both surfaces oozed with blood. I followed the colon forward to its junction with the small intestine and then immediately lost free bowel.

"Oh, Sonja, I'm so sorry. This looks hopeless."

"What do you think happened?" she asked quietly.

"It appears that she ended up with a tear in her suspensory apparatus somewhere back here." I indicated the area near the junction of the small and large bowel where everything seemed to coalesce into a welded, confused mess. "The tear must have happened when she got hit by the car; the bowel slowly worked its way through and ended up trapped."

"Well, why wouldn't our vet have been able to pick that up?" Sonja asked, struggling with tears.

"Like Siggy said, Trixie didn't seem to be in pain at the time she was first presented, and there probably was no reason to suspect it. Even if she was a bit tender on abdominal palpation, most vets—me included—would have just observed her."

I struggled with the entanglement in a desperate attempt to work at least some portions of the bowel free. The surfaces were glued tight.

Sonja burst into tears and rushed from the surgery. I looked at Doris and shrugged my shoulders. I couldn't believe what I had found. I could tell from Doris's face that she was wishing she were home puttering around her kitchen.

After ten minutes of struggling with the mess of bowel, I approached Sonja in the waiting room. She had pulled off her mask and cap and sat with her head in her hands. She glanced up at me. Her eyes were red, and black streaks of mascara stained her face.

"I'm sorry. I can't begin to straighten things out." I stood helplessly with my bloody hands clutched in front of me. "If I thought there was even a hope, I'd suggest we close her up and take her to the veterinary teaching hospital at Pullman."

"I know," Sonja said. "Can I use your phone?" She marched to the reception desk. "I better get hold of Siggy."

Trixie's chest rose and fell rhythmically as if she were patiently waiting for me to correct the problem and wake her up. I peered down at the jumbled concretion of guts. I had been certain that this was going to be something simple. I tried one last time to work my fingers into the tangle—to pry something free.

I could hear the Wittmosers' veterinarian now. "Why didn't he just straighten it out?" Why not, indeed? I gave up as blood oozed from the surfaces of the bowel I had tried to separate. I was frustrated enough at not being able to correct the situation, but what was worse, I had no sensible explanation for what had caused such adhesions to form.

I reached forward in search of the duodenum and the pancreas. Had there been enzymes leaking into the abdominal cavity? There had been no indication of infection or perforation of the bowel. The white blood cell counts had been normal on all the tests that had been run in Calgary.

"We leave it up to you, Doctor."

The woman's voice cut through my internal rhetoric. I turned toward the doorway of the surgery. Sonja's face was downcast.

"We both agree that we don't want her to suffer," she added hesitantly. "She's always been such an active, happy dog. She absolutely loved our new home at Crawford Bay, and now…"

I stared numbly at the jumbled mass of bowel before me. What a way to meet new clients. If only I could magically break down all those adhesions. The valves on the anesthetic machine rattled as Trixie took another deep breath.

"I know what I'd do if she were my dog."

"You'd put her to sleep?" Sonja prompted.

I nodded.

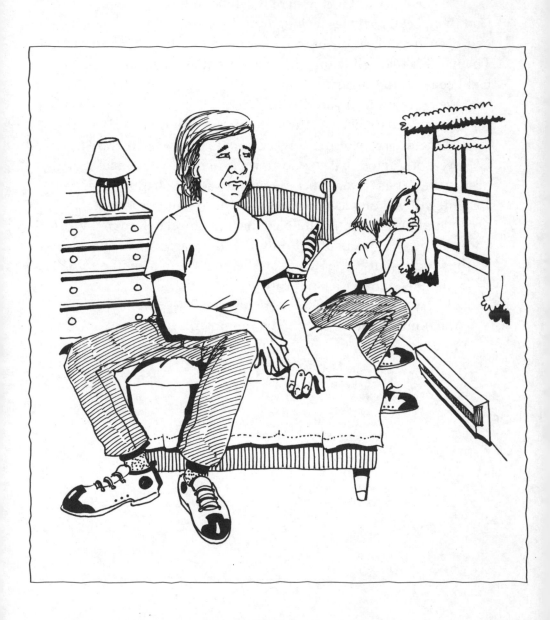

Moving On

I sat in the office shuffling through the reports of recently returned post-mortem results. One would have concluded from the number of Tsolum Farms files that the Hurfords had a higher than normal death loss with their herd. But that wasn't the case at all—Herb was just diligent about knowing what was going on at his farm. As a matter of fact, there was hardly a critter that died on the property that he didn't request a post-mortem for. Three more cows had died of this horrendous mastitis.

I had gotten to the point of apoplexy when either the Hurford name or Tsolum Farms appeared on the day page. I was sick to death of the seemingly insurmountable problem there. I could only imagine how Herb and his sons were feeling each time they had to call me. It was so frustrating for me to be unable to help— to be unable to come up with a firm diagnosis. There had to be an answer that I had not yet detected somewhere in all this gibberish.

I thumbed through the lab results from May 28. The description of the samples from cow #93 was so familiar. I could almost recite word for word the pathologist's comments—the medical terminology that described tissue death from one end of the cow to the other. I had been so certain that first day that the bacteriology results would be immediately conclusive. We just had to be dealing with an exceptionally hot *E. coli* or klebsiella mastitis. To my knowledge, nothing else produced such a devastating mastitis.

How could they have drawn a blank and cultured nothing significant from all those hunks of dead meat I sent to the lab? All they had grown was an organism called *Bacillus cereus*, a bug that was considered an obvious contaminant.

I shook my head in disgust and flipped over the page. I remembered how my hackles had gone up when I first read that comment. Number 93 had been such a strange case that I had been extra careful when I did the post-mortem, determined not to miss a thing. I had bagged the fresh pieces the moment I cut them free from the cow's body—how could they have been contaminated? Another vet reading this report would wonder whether I had marinated each sample in a pound of dirt.

The second report was of #113, the cow that had followed on the heels of #93. Marcie and I had attended her shortly after the raft race. The histological description for that poor cow was exactly the same as the first one—tremendous inflammation with massive tissue death in all the samples examined. I followed the report to its conclusion. There had been no growth at all on any of her samples —hard to believe of specimens that were taken from an animal that died of such an overwhelming infection. Maybe the causative organism was just hard to grow. Maybe the massive levels of antibiotics that I had used had provided a residue effect powerful enough to neutralize the bug before it got to the laboratory.

I thought back to the contamination theory. Hell, if there had been room for introduction of stray organisms, it would have been with this post-mortem. It had poured with rain when I was out there with #113. I had sloshed around in mud up to the top of my boots and had water running down the crack of my arse. I came close to miring my poor car at the edge of the cornfield that day. Even under those conditions, I made damn sure that there was nothing but the cow parts in those sample bags.

I flipped the report over. The next submission was a list of ten cows that I had sent for culture. All of them had been samples collected and frozen from cows that had been treated for clinical mastitis over a three-week period. Four of them had produced no growth, three had grown *Staph aureus*, two of them *Strep agalactia*, and one had been positive for *Bacillus cereus*.

What was with this *Bacillus cereus*, anyway? I had never heard mention of the organism before, and now I was getting it in one sample after the other. The bacteriologist's cryptic note was: "Contaminant." But was it really? Sometimes those ivory tower pathologists really annoyed me. For guys who got to sit in their fancy labs with nice clean white smocks, they were quick to judge those of us who were slogging in the trenches.

I grabbed the reports I'd been reading and dialled the number indicated. Damn! All I got was a recording giving the lab's hours. I glanced at the day page. It figured—Saturday morning. Amazing how one day seemed like the next in this job.

I was getting antsy. The breakthrough I was hoping for was slow in coming. Knowing that I had two more samples at the provincial lab waiting for processing was like having two lottery tickets in my wallet. As slim as the chances might be to win the jackpot, there was always the hope that one of these days I'd get lucky.

Ten days ago I had mailed the samples from #88. She had died like all of the others, and I had sent pounds more flesh: mammary tissue, lymph nodes, spleen, liver, kidneys—you name it.

Another cow, #111, was literally hanging on to life by the skin of her teat. I had collected a sample of fluid from three affected quarters of her udder and started incubating it immediately on blood agar culture media with the hope that something would grow. Number 111 had literally refused to die, even though those affected quarters had turned into a rotting mass. When I was there for my weekly herd health session the day before, she was actually beginning to pick at her feed despite the fact that great hunks of decaying matter dangled from the remains of her udder.

I was kicking myself now for not phoning the lab on Thursday or Friday. When I had called on Tuesday, only the results of the histology on the first cow were complete. They had been just like the last ones—necrosis, necrosis, and more necrosis. This bug killed tissue like nothing I had ever seen.

Doris hadn't had time to get the mail on Friday and promised to pick it up this morning just in case they had completed a report. The door opened out front. It was 8:15—that must be her.

"Dave. You in here?"

"Back here, John…Did you wet the bed? Isn't it a bit early for you to be up on a Saturday morning?"

The boy appeared at the doorway all dressed up with a white shirt and tie. "Have to be at work soon, but I wanted a chance to talk to you."

"Sure thing." I put the lab reports aside. "What's up?"

"I've got a chance to do a sheet metal apprenticeship in Calgary, Dave." John presented the matter-of-fact statement as a question. He glanced timidly toward me.

"I need to do something with my life. I know I could stay working at Super-Valu until Brian graduates, but that'll put me behind two years. I might just get stuck there like some of the other guys. Do you remember what you told me when I started work? You told me there was nothing wrong with being a meat cutter, but don't stick with it just because it's a job and it looks like good money. You told me I can be whatever I want to be."

I looked into the boy's earnest face. In his own roundabout way, he was asking my permission to leave Creston. Staring into the teen's perplexed blue eyes, I could see how difficult this was for him. Why should an eighteen-year-old carry such a burden?

"When would you start?"

"I have to be there for the fifteenth of August."

I was struggling to keep from showing my emotions. After all, only last month Brian and I had endured John's graduation ceremony. Although I had joked with him that I was sure my butt cheeks would be numb forever, I wouldn't have missed it for anything. As boring as those sessions could be, I was wiping tears from my eyes as I watched the tall lad stride jauntily across the stage to receive his diploma. I smiled, remembering how his long curly locks poked from beneath his box cap.

It seemed like only yesterday that he had appeared at the office with his younger brother after Brian's dog, Boots, had been run over by a car. Had it really been three years? I couldn't have foreseen how the boys would become such an integral part of my life.

I was so proud of John and his desire to make something of himself. How many kids started out as wards of child welfare and cultivated the drive for success that this boy had? Working two and three jobs at a time, he always had a goal to accomplish. First, it was nice clothes, and then it was his beater, the Fiat. Now it was a new career. I wondered what it was that made some people so determined to succeed. From the very beginning John was loath to take anything he hadn't earned. The first time the boys worked for me, they hadn't eaten the entire day, yet John insisted they were full. I could still see the look in his brother's eyes when John turned down the offer of lunch. I chuckled at the thought of how voraciously they had eaten when John finally relented. Those salami sandwiches had literally disappeared like props in a Houdini magic act.

"Where will you live?" I asked quietly. I was struggling to keep the tone of my voice upbeat.

"For the first little while, with Vince. He was good to us when we lived in Calgary. I told you about him—he was Mom's boyfriend before she started drinking all the time and chasing after drugs."

I nodded. The boys' stories stuck in my mind—of waking to the sound of wild parties, of strange men with bags of pills coming and going from their derelict apartment at all hours of the day and night. Vince had apparently been there for the boys during those trying times.

I smiled at him. "I'm sure you'll do just fine, John." I looked away so he couldn't see the tears that welled. Lug sensed the anguish in my voice and presented his head for a scratch. After a long pause, I stared into the dog's big brown eyes and blurted, "I'll miss you around here."

"Yeah, I'll miss you—and Martha, too," John mumbled.

We both stared at the floor in opposite corners of the room as I struggled to overcome the urge to take him in my arms and give him a hug. I ran my hands over Lug's back and scratched him over the base of his tail.

After a long pause, I asked, "What about Brian?"

"I told him last night." The boy's eyes were rivetted on the floor. "He never said another word all night. Before that, he was babbling away about meeting his buddies and going down to the river. He hasn't left his room since."

"Maybe we better go pick him up."

I could only surmise how troubling John's decision would be to Brian. With his mother gone, he was almost totally dependent on his brother for parenting, for direction, for hope that the pair had some sort of future. Although Martha and I had become family to both of them, there was no doubt in my mind that it was John Brian couldn't do without.

John wiped his eyes, then turned sheepishly in my direction. "I gotta be at work in ten minutes."

"Okay. I think I better stop around to see him."

John nodded and headed for the door. Just then it opened and Doris bustled in.

"Good morning, John…and how are you today?"

"Pretty good," he mumbled. He squeezed past her and ran off down the street without looking back.

My sidekick looked perplexed as she set her purse on the counter. "Is everything all right?" she queried in her motherly fashion.

"Not really." Sometimes I wished that my face could be less expressive.

"What's up?"

"John's leaving. He's taken a position in Calgary as a sheet metal apprentice."

Doris gave me a knowing look. "He's a go-getter, that boy…We'll miss him around here."

"Yeah," I mumbled pathetically.

She handed me a stack of mail. "There's two in there from the lab…I hope they're the ones you're looking for."

I grabbed the letters and impatiently tore the first one open. It was a report on some serum samples from Partington cows that I had sent in several weeks back. Without even reading the results, I tore open the second one—Tsolum Farms. I rushed through the reams of histological description in search of the bacteriological results.

A shiver ran up my spine when I read it—*Bacillus cereus*. I paid particular attention to the pathologist's comments: "Although *Bacillus cereus* is not known to be an aggressive pathogen in the cause of mastitis, in this case it is unlikely to be a contaminant as it was cultured from the mammary tissue, a lymph node, and also the liver."

I sat numbly trying to absorb the impact of his conclusion. If this one was *not* a contaminant, then neither were the others. I dug through the earlier reports—each case had been worked by a different pathologist.

So the smoking gun had been there all along. If this were the real culprit, then the tremendous tissue death made sense. The only other bacillus species I knew of was *Bacillus anthracis*, the organism that caused anthrax. Everyone on the street knew how devastating that organism could be.

"Were they the ones you were waiting for?" Doris asked.

I nodded, feeling a brief respite from my discontent. "I'm going out to Martha's to have a talk with Brian."

"Just remember that you have a ten o'clock appointment with Richls. He's got a cow that hasn't been milking out properly on one of her teats, so make sure you've got all your instruments."

I was apprehensive as I approached the old two-storey house in Riverview. This wasn't going to be easy. And I knew Martha would be upset as well. She was such a motherly sort, and as the boys' foster parent, she had seen them through those difficult early days after their own mother disappeared. I knocked on the kitchen door. The tall, dark-haired woman opened it and invited me in. I engaged her hazel eyes.

"How's Brian?"

"I haven't seen the boy all morning." She glanced at the stairway that led to his upstairs bedroom. "I knocked on the door and asked him if he wanted breakfast, but he told me he wasn't hungry." She kneaded the tea towel in her hands as if it were bread dough and said mournfully, "There's something wrong when that boy won't eat."

Our eyes met again. "John told you his plans?" I asked.

Martha turned away from me to the sink full of dishes and nodded. "He filled me in this morning at breakfast."

"I'm going up to talk to Brian." I spoke to the woman's back as she chucked her towel aside and immersed her hands in the soapy water.

I stopped at the first door at the top of the stairs and knocked softly. "Brian?" There was an uncomfortable silence as I waited for acknowledgement. "Can I come in?"

"Yeah," he finally replied.

I opened the door and stooped to enter. Although he usually made some wisecrack about my not being designed for his room, today he said nothing. He lay stretched full-length on his bed, his face buried in the pillow, his right hand resting awkwardly on the top of his head.

"You all right?"

"Yeah." His monosyllabic reply was less than convincing.

Tired of stooping in the low-ceilinged room, I sat on the edge of the bed. "John told me his plans this morning."

There was no reply.

"Look at me, Brian."

Damn! Although I spoke softly, my voice had more of an edge than I meant it to. The boy slowly turned in my direction. He deliberately raised himself, using both arms as if doing a push-up. Halfway up, he scrunched the pillow to cover the wet spot his tears had left on the linen case. His expression was one of anguish and uncertainty.

"Things'll work out all right."

His normally vibrant blue eyes were red from crying. "What'll I do without John?" His voice trailed off.

"It'll be hard at first. I know you'll miss him…We all will. He's right, though. If he stays working at Super-Valu, he may just get stuck there. You know John wants to try something different."

He looked away from me. Shifting himself to the other side of the bed, he stared out the tiny window. "Do you think I could go with him?"

I stared numbly at the back of the boy's head. I felt myself being drawn into his vortex of gloom—I could be losing not one but both of my boys!

"Is that what you want?" My voice wavered.

Brian nodded slowly.

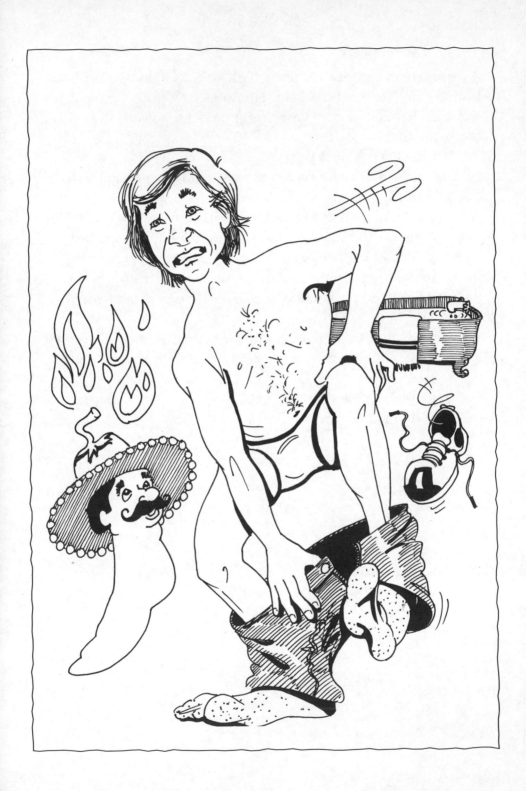

Hot Stuff

"You guys really don't think I can cook, do you?"

John smiled meekly and took a playful poke at Brian. "You make real good peanut butter sandwiches…doesn't he, Bri?"

I feigned a look of disdain. "I cooked all the time when I was going to college…and some of it tasted good."

John nodded to placate me.

"Well, why don't you guys come over for supper tonight, and then we'll take in a movie. I'll make up some of my world-famous chili and prove to you what a great cook I am."

I ducked through the doorway, descended the stairs, and left the house. I had to get out of there. Seeing the boys' room without all the pictures on the wall, without all their personal effects, was just too final. Martha was kneeling beside the walkway digging with a hand trowel in her begonias. I was about to ask her if she had any tips on making good chili when she spoke.

"Hard to believe they're leaving us, isn't it?"

"Sure is."

I didn't want to face the fact that by this time tomorrow the boys would be gone from my daily life. All the time I had spent dreading this moment had made me no more ready for it than when John had broken the news last month.

Martha smiled gently. "I've had a lot of children come and go. They're all special in some way, but I can't think of any that have touched me more than they have."

John came out of the house with a cardboard box full of clothing. I followed him down the walk.

"Have you got any room left in there?" I rushed ahead to open the door of the little red Fiat and rearranged some boxes so that he could squeeze in his burden. "Is this heap going to get you guys out there?"

The boy gave me his usual broad grin. "You bet—she's never let me down yet."

John was reorganizing his treasures on the back seat as I left. I felt strangely melancholic as I stuck my arm out the window in salute and pulled onto the roadway. Where had the time gone? It seemed like just yesterday that I had been teaching the boy to drive, and now he was about to steer his old jalopy right out of my life.

I headed down the road toward Creston. In a way, I was envious of the boys. Why should I have to stay here and face the music when I could drive into the sunset, too? What had become of the storybook notion that I could save every critter I touched and make money hand over fist for every producer that used my services?

I was still struggling to make sense of the mastitis outbreak at Tsolum Farms. When the milk samples from 111 came back positive for *Bacillus cereus*, there was no question it had to be considered the causative agent of the outbreak. But that didn't explain why this relatively unknown species of bacillus had chosen Tsolum Farms in Creston, British Columbia, to make its debut as a pathogen.

I had left no stone unturned that I could think of. The local electrician had spent days looking for abnormalities in the power supply that could be causing problems in the milking parlour. The company that manufactured and supplied the equipment had been through the facility from one end to the other ruling out mechanical problems. I had spent hours watching the guys during milking to see if bad technique could be contributing. I had even cultured everyone's hands in search of a carrier and gotten them to milk with rubber gloves. What had I overlooked?

Hours on the telephone talking to experts at the provincial lab and at the veterinary college in Saskatoon had been unproductive. The one suggestion that offered a glimmer of hope had come from this morning's talk with Jeremy Greenfield, the bacteriologist at the lab. He suggested the possibility of preparing a bacterin from several of the isolates that could be utilized as a vaccine for the remaining cows. He had apparently had success using it against some strains of E. coli and thought it might be helpful here. I'd give Hurfords a call about that option in the morning.

Parking in the Super-Valu lot, I ran into the store. I didn't have much time to get supper ready if we were going to make the seven o'clock show at the Tivoli Theatre. I rushed quickly around the aisles and arrived at the till with a two-pound package of hamburger, a container of chili powder, a bag of onions, a loaf of Italian bread, and a gallon of chocolate ice cream.

I caught myself looking toward the meat section in search of John. I had shopped at the store regularly since the boy started working here. It would be strange not seeing him running around in the back keeping the shelves in order.

Lug watched expectantly as I peeled the cellophane wrapper from the hamburger.

"You think you need some, do you?"

I pinched a crumble from the end of the pack and dropped it into his waiting mouth. He gobbled it without even tasting it and stood waiting hopefully with tail wagging.

I broke up the meat in the pot with a fork and turned up the heat. At the kitchen sink, I chopped a couple of onions and a green pepper. This felt good. I hadn't cooked anything in ages and had sort of forgotten how much fun it could be. I stirred the beef and spent the next five minutes poking away at the lumps to break them down. Throwing in the veggies, I turned down the heat and covered the pot. There was something reassuring about the sound of supper sizzling on the stove.

I wasn't sure what was playing at the Tiv tonight, but it didn't really matter. I was going to spend this last night together with the boys—come hell or high water.

I hurried downstairs and made a quick round of my patients. The Labrador retriever that I had spayed earlier in the morning was up and rooting through the bars for attention.

"Hey, sweetie…you're looking good."

I rubbed her nose between the upright rails and proceeded down the line to Cali. A beautiful calico cat, Cali had come up just a little slow when trying to outrun a pickup truck. She had rallied well from her injuries, and I was sure that we would soon be able to pin her fractured hind leg. I stroked the cat as she huddled with her eyes closed and her splinted limb held uncomfortably to the side.

"There's a girl, Cali. You're such a pretty kitty, aren't you?"

She shoved her head into the palm of my hand and rubbed it repeatedly. Her entire body vibrated as her larynx ground out a deep-throated purr. I extended her foreleg and massaged gently over the area where a catheter penetrated her skin. It was still in the vein and the fluids were running with a steady drip, drip, drip.

Halfway up the stairs I was greeted by the aroma of my supper cooking. It was going to be great. I stirred the pot and scooped up a forkful. Blowing on the steaming morsel, I took a hesitant bite. Not bad, but it sure needed something. I shook in first salt, then pepper: better, but still in need. I thrashed around in the cupboard for garlic powder. I was sure I had some here somewhere. I added a jumbo tin of kidney beans and one of tomatoes, then punched out the large hole from the can of chili powder and shook some in. I grabbed a spoon and tried the sauce—it was a long way from what I was looking for. Where was that garlic powder? I plowed through the shelves one more time. Damn! When had I used it last?

I turned down the heat on the stove and dashed out the door. I was down the street and turning into the Super-Valu in no time flat. I rushed around the store. Grabbing a container of garlic powder and a little net bag of real garlic, I hurried through the checkout.

On my way home past the Tivoli, I noticed that *Papillon* was playing. I enjoyed Steve McQueen and had heard that this movie was well worth watching. I was really looking forward to this night out with the boys.

By the time I huffed up the stairs and entered the apartment, I was castigating myself for not buying mushrooms. It wasn't as if I hadn't had the opportunity. Hell, I had walked by them twice and even noticed how fresh they looked. I added the garlic, chopping one clove at a time. I was peeling a fifth when I hesitated. I didn't want to get too carried away. I'd let this simmer for a bit and then see.

I took a quick run downstairs. Cali seemed comfortable and her IV was fine. I could still see those mushrooms in my mind's eye—they would sure have made the difference in the chili.

I lifted the lid and checked my goulash again. Dipping the spoon into the concoction, I raised it to my nose. It smelled richer with the garlic. I tasted. Better…but a long way from what I was imagining. I glanced at my watch—just a few minutes to five. I still had time. One more trip wouldn't kill me…I needed the exercise anyway.

I had filled a paper bag with mushrooms and was heading for the checkout when I spied a display of jalapeño peppers. That might be the missing link, the zing my chili needed. I had never used them before, but it wouldn't hurt to give a small one a try.

Lug greeted me at the top of the stairs, his tail in full wag. He was more than a little upset by the fact that he hadn't been invited to go with me on all these excursions and was convinced I was up to something. I gave him a hurried pat and rumpled his ears, anxious to get all these ingredients into the chili and give them time to simmer.

I rinsed the mushrooms, sliced them, and stirred them into the pot. I tasted the juice. Not bad at all—maybe I should leave well enough alone. I hesitated for a moment, then returned to the sink and cut through the little green pepper. It was only three inches long and couldn't really make that much difference. I sliced it down the middle and chopped it finely. I thought about just adding half, but it looked like such a piddly amount. I chopped the remainder into tiny pieces and scraped the whole thing into the mixture. I stirred it well, cleaned up the mess at the sink, and gave my hands a cursory rinse. For better or worse, supper was ready.

I headed to the bathroom for a quick leak. Looking at myself in the mirror, I ran my hand over my cheeks. I was getting as bad as Pop with my five-o'clock shadow—I could remember when I stayed nice and smooth all day. I unzipped my fly and got down to business. I hoped the chili passed the next taste test. The boys would be here any time.

I was on my way back to the stove when I realized I was in trouble. My face was suddenly aglow and my cheeks were burning. Within seconds I was digging at my crotch. I beat a hasty retreat to the bathroom and peered in the mirror. Both sides of my face were a blotchy red. I grabbed a washcloth and scrubbed madly at my face. My God, I was on fire!

I kicked off my shoes and tore at my jeans. My pant legs hung up and I pranced wildly from one side to the other in a mad dance to be free of them. They finally released and I flicked my jeans into the corner. I pulled off my underpants, smeared soap on the cloth, and scrubbed vigorously at my groin.

"AAAAhhhhh!"

All I managed to do was spread the area of concern south to my backside. I raced to the tub to start the water running, submersed my hands in the flow, and rubbed them anxiously back and forth on the bar of Ivory soap. Terrified to touch myself anywhere, I plunked my butt into the shallow water at the far end of the tub and began splashing frantically. I couldn't believe the intensity of the pain. The cool waters seemed to moderate the fires of hell. I kept scrubbing, and finally with tentative strokes, massaged my face with suds.

It was working. The burning sensation on my cheeks was beginning to subside. I scrubbed a towel with soap and attacked the inferno in my groin. As the pain diminished, I lay back and sloshed water over my private parts. Reluctantly, I eased myself from the water and dried off. I gingerly stepped into my underwear and pulled on my pants and shirt.

What had I done to my culinary creation? If a little bit of juice from that fool pepper could cause so much trauma, what had its flesh done to my chili? I hoped I hadn't ruined everything. My one opportunity to impress the boys with my cooking skills, and I had to pull a fool stunt like this. I glanced at my watch—no time to start over.

I carefully removed the pot lid and eyed the concoction. It looked great, and those mushrooms definitely gave it an appearance of richness. I bent down and took a sniff—it smelled simply wonderful. I didn't know what I was expecting—maybe that it would knock me over like the vapours from some toxic waste dump.

I stirred happily. Cooking must definitely break that stuff down. There was no doubt about it—this was going to be good. I spooned up a sample consisting of a mushroom, some meat, and a couple of beans. I blew on it until I was sure that it was just the right temperature, cautiously chewed, and swallowed.

It was a bit hot. I could tell that from the outset, but nothing compared to what I'd imagined. I was going for a second spoonful when it hit me. It was a searing heat from the back of my mouth to the depth of my esophagus. I took two or three quick breaths, then ran to the sink. I turned on the cold water tap and opened my mouth under it. Gulping down the water, I attempted to dilute the heat. If it worked on the outside, surely it would help on the inside.

Damn! Why hadn't I added the pepper a bit at a time like any reasonable person would do? Now the whole supper was ruined. I peered at my watch. I could still add more ingredients to try and dilute it. The Super-Valu was closed, but Paul's Superette would be open.

I closed the door in Lug's face and thumped down the stairs two at a time. At the corner store, my mouth was still on fire—surely there would be some way of nullifying the toxin. I grabbed two more cans each of kidney beans and tomatoes. At the till I added a bag of licorice.

I raced down the street munching voraciously on the strawberry twists. I was happy to see that the boys had yet to arrive and there was still an opportunity for me to save face. Lug was wagging uncertainly as I opened the door. I had consumed half the bag of candy on the way home, and the burn had faded to a mild sense of irritation. Oh, how I hoped that dilution was the solution.

I activated the can opener and quickly emptied more beans and tomatoes into the pot. Stirring with my fingers crossed, I silently prayed that I had solved the problem. I filled a spoon with sauce and gingerly raised it to my lips.

Please. Please. Please…Yes!

That had definitely tamed it down. I waited a second and was just about to try a spoonful with a couple of mushrooms when it hit me. Was it still just the residual from last time? Maybe I was sensitized to the burning sensation and just a little bit could get me going. I tried the second spoonful.

Oh, my God!

I ran for the opener and attacked the remaining cans. Just a bit more dilution would be the answer. My pot was filled to the brim. I poured some into a plastic bowl and stuck it in the fridge.

I filled Lug's dish with kibble and dumped some chili on top. "Looks like you'll be getting a treat for a few days, boy."

He wolfed down a mouthful, then flopped down in the corner.

"Oh Lord, is it that bad?"

I dumped in another can of kidney beans and a small can of stewed tomatoes. I was just stirring it in when Lug's ears perked up. The bottom door opened and the boys came thundering up the stairs.

"That's okay, Lug. It's just the guys...Go eat your supper." I glared at the dog as he wagged his tail and went to greet them.

"Well, I hope you're hungry!" I boomed with far more aplomb than the occasion demanded.

"We're starved," John assured me. "Bri was out visiting all day, and I just finished doing an oil change...Never even stopped for lunch."

"I forgot to ask you, do you like your chili hot?"

"Sure," John assured me, "hot's good. Mom used to make it pretty hot."

"Just make yourselves comfortable, guys. Supper's almost ready."

I glared at Lug again as he wandered into the living room with the guests—ungrateful mutt. That's the last time he could expect a treat from me.

The boys seemed subdued. Brian clicked on the television while John stood at the doorway and talked a bit about what it would be like back in Alberta after three years away.

"Are you going to Calgary for a bit too, Brian?" I raised my voice to get through to him over the droning of a talk show.

The boy shrugged. "Yeah, I'll maybe stay with John a few days before Vince takes me down to Taber."

"Taber's quite a ways from Calgary," I began. "I thought you wanted to be close to John...Could you live with Vince?"

"I could, maybe..." The boy gazed at the television. Both John and I studied him as he squirmed uncomfortably. "Mr. Blair at social services said that the Johnsons called him and asked if I wanted to live with them."

I nodded. "He mentioned that to me."

"They have a farm with lots of animals and stuff," the boy

mumbled. There was a total lack of enthusiasm in his voice.

"Vince said he could stay with us," John added hopefully.

"How do you know these people?" I pried.

"He used to work with Vince," John offered. "We went to their place for two summers in a row when we were still living in Calgary."

"So it's a farm?"

Brian continued gazing at the television, seemingly content that John had taken over the talking.

"Yeah," John responded. "But not a very big one."

"What kind of animals, Brian?" The boy stared vacantly ahead.

"Pigs, cows, and chickens," John responded after a moment of silence.

"What are the people like?"

"They're okay," Brian mumbled.

I headed back to the kitchen. "Just remember, Brian, you always have a home with me or with Martha…You've got a lot of friends here."

The boy nodded.

I set the table while they stared at the television. Lug came back from the living room, took a few hesitant licks at his food, made a couple of slow turns, and plunked down with his nose inches from his dish. I was not impressed. The least he could have done was give it a good second chance.

I sliced the loaf of Italian bread and set it on the table, then flipped a dozen pickles into a bowl.

"Okay, let's eat!" The boys rushed into the kitchen and took a place at the table. "Load up, guys."

John heaped several spoonfuls onto his plate and passed the ladle to Brian.

"Smells great, Dave."

"Thanks…Hope it tastes as good."

I took my plate to the stove for a single scoop. John dug in heartily. He had taken a couple of forkfuls and still seemed ready for more. My attempt at diluting the fiery stew must have done the trick. Brian was more conservative—he was still working on his first mouthful.

I sat down and forked a nice big hunk of mushroom into my mouth. Not bad—I had definitely diluted the problem considerably. Heartened, I took a mouthful of the entire concoction—meat, beans, peppers, sauce—and was just about certain that I had the problem licked when John set down his fork and reached for a slice of bread. Quickly buttering it, he stuffed his mouth full and chewed diligently. Brian took a long drink of water before voraciously attacking a pickle.

It was only after I swallowed that I got a true appreciation for the power of the jalapeño. I bravely took a second and third mouthful. Although not as intense as before, the burn was continuous. I was trying to convince myself that the tingle was only due to my previous sensitization when Brian and John simultaneously reached for another piece of bread.

"Pass the pickles, will you, Bri?" He speared three baby dills and lined them up in a row along the edge of his plate.

"Hot enough for you guys? You told me you liked it hot, so if you want me to warm it up a bit, I could add some more chili pepper."

"No," Brian stammered, "no, it's hot enough for me."

He drained his glass, and after a quick look at John, hurried to the sink for a refill.

"Mine, too," John insisted, passing his glass to his brother.

I continued eating as if this chili was my favourite dish. Spooning a mound onto my bread, I took a bite. Brian mimicked me, thinking that maybe I had come up with a magic way of toning down the heat.

"Eat up, guys. I've got a gallon of chocolate ice cream in the freezer."

Brian began shovelling in earnest. Within moments he had his plate clean and had finished his water.

"Need a refill, Bri? There's lots there."

"Ah…no thanks, Dave. I'm full to the brim."

"How you doing, John…a little more?"

"No thanks, Dave. I'm doin' good."

"Do you mind if I get my ice cream, Dave?" asked Brian.

"No, go ahead."

He popped another pickle into his mouth and rushed to the fridge. Within seconds he had retrieved the frozen tub and was filling a soup bowl with ice cream. Before Brian got back to the table, the first heaping spoonful of the chocolate treat was on the way to his gullet. He closed his eyes as if savouring the relief.

John grimaced as he watched his brother tackling the impressive mound of chocolate. Grabbing another piece of bread, he attacked his plate with a vengeance. Although he was getting close to polishing it off, he was slowing down. He swallowed the last heel of bread and poked with his fork to spread the remaining chili as thinly as possible around the plate.

I stood up and took it from him. "Are you sure you wouldn't like a bit more?"

"No thanks, Dave…stuffed to the gills." He was already on his way to the counter to dish up his ice cream. "You want some, Dave?" he asked, digging mercilessly into the bucket.

"If there's any left," I said.

While Brian and John ate their dessert, they immersed themselves in a rerun episode of *Gilligan's Island*.

With the boys preoccupied, I was able to scoop more than my share of the cool treat. As the burning sensation subsided, it was replaced with the uncomfortable feeling of an overdose of ice cream.

"Are you guys ready?"

"Just a second," Brian insisted. "This show's almost over."

I sat down and watched as Gilligan did battle with a huge gorilla that had Mary Ann in its clutches.

"It's almost seven, you guys," I pestered, "that's when the show starts."

"There's ten or fifteen minutes of previews," Brian countered. "We got lots of time."

I was just ushering the boys out the door when the phone rang. I tensed immediately and found myself resisting the need to answer it. It sometimes seemed as if people were watching so they could interrupt me the moment I started having fun.

John gave me a knowing look. "You better take it."

I smiled meekly at him and picked up the phone. "Creston Veterinary Clinic."

"Oh, glad I was able to catch you, Dave. It's Bernie Riehl calling. I've got a cow that just pushed out her womb."

I took a deep breath and looked sadly at the boys, who were standing outside the door monitoring the conversation.

"She's looking pretty rough," Bernie said after a moment of silence. "Dave...are you there?"

The boys watched me expectantly.

"I'll be out there shortly, Bernie."

I put down the phone. Brian hung his head and sank to his knees to give Lug a hug.

"Sorry, guys, you'll have to go it alone." I passed John a twenty. "I was looking forward to this as much as you were."

Brian focused his big blue eyes on me. "That's okay, Dave, we know what it's like. Guess we wouldn't have met you if you just worked regular hours. Bootsie got run over on a weekend, remember? We worked together on him all day."

He hugged Lug one last time, and he and John headed down the stairs. They both turned when they reached the landing and waved half-heartedly. I raised my hand in return and then let it fall onto Lug's head. The door rattled shut and the boys were gone from my life.

I collapsed into the recliner. Lug rested his head on my lap and gazed up at me with knowing eyes. Why, when I tried my hardest to make things go right, did they always go awry? *I try to make a special dinner, and I almost poison them. I ask them to go to a movie, and I send them off alone.*

Such was the life of a country vet—certainly, such was the life of *this* country vet. I got up and prowled the room. I was sure going to miss those boys. Their frequent appearances in my life had provided such a welcome change of pace. Suddenly, I felt very much alone in my little world. I picked up the phone and dialled the number that I now knew by heart.

"Hello, Marcie? It's Dave calling…Sounds like I've got an interesting case if you want to tag along. It's a prolapsed uterus."

She was as keen as ever. I had become increasingly more dependent upon my student for assistance. She was good with critters, she was observant, and she had an avid interest in learning all she could. She was also insistent that I call her at any time during her off-hours if there happened to be an unusual case. Fascinated with clinical medicine, she had only taken the summer job with the government to earn enough money to help her through her final year at veterinary college.

We first treated the huge Holstein cow for the calcium deficiency that predisposed a dairy cow to prolapse, then worked on the uterus until we finally had it pushed back in. By the time the last of the pink flesh had disappeared through the cow's vagina and I had sutured her up, we were both soaked and bloody from head to foot. There was certainly nothing prissy about this girl.

After cleaning up as well as we could in Bernie's milk house, we headed back to Creston.

"Did you hear any more from the lab about Tsolum Farms?" she asked.

I sighed. If there had ever been a series of cases designed to dissuade a fledgling vet from venturing into large animal practice, this was it. Thank heavens for the opportunity to show her a few cases like this one at the Riehls, where a vet could actually make a difference.

"I had a conference call with several pathologists from the provincial lab this morning. They don't know what to think of the situation. They're all on the bandwagon about *Bacillus cereus* being the cause of our problems, because now it's showing up on some farms down in the Fraser Valley. They're going to try to come up with a vaccine for Herb's cows. It's sort of scary to even think of injecting that crap into a healthy animal, but Jeremy Greenfield thinks it might help. I guess he just prepares a culture from a few different samples and kills it with formalin."

She wrinkled her brow. "Wouldn't want any of that stuff injected into me," she said with a shiver. "I'll never forget the poor cow I saw at Hurfords…Will they try it on mice or something?"

"I never thought to ask, but I will. Herb'll probably come up with the same question. Jeremy said they'll want me to try it on a few test cows first."

I pulled up to her front door in Erickson. "Well, thanks for calling me," she said. "That was quite the case."

I smiled as I watched her slosh her way up the sidewalk, looking very much like an axe-murderer on a spree. The more I saw of this woman, the more I was convinced that she was going to be a good veterinarian. A caring attitude and the desire to just dig in— no matter what the circumstances—were real assets to a rural practice like mine. I wondered if she'd actually consider Creston as a destination after her graduation.

I sighed. She would soon be gone, too—first the boys, now Marcie.

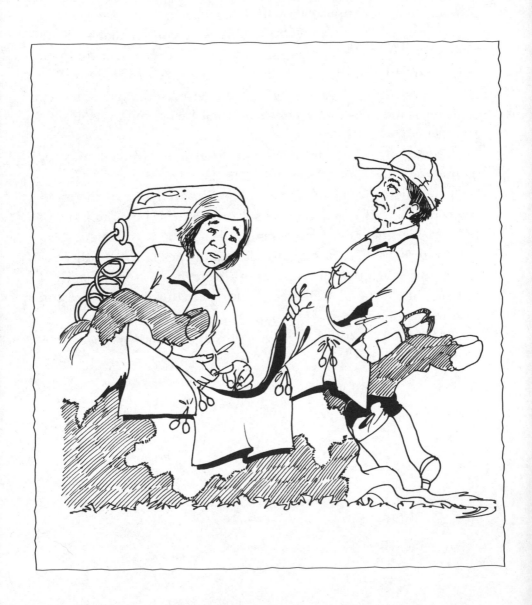

House of Beauty

"Dave, you have to do something about your hair!"

Doris kept close track of the length of my mane, preferring crewcuts to the long, unkempt style of the day.

"Let me phone Tom and see if he can squeeze you in this morning. Partingtons just cancelled their herd health inspection."

I stooped to the lab mirror and peered at my reflection. I was looking a bit scruffier than usual, and my sideburns were creeping further and further down my cheeks.

"Okay. Give him a call and see if he has a moment."

A trip to the Manell House of Beauty was always an experience. As Creston's only openly gay couple, the boys were considered a bit of an oddity in our sleepy little town. Although I first got to know them through their toy poodle, Belinda, I became hooked on their antics and now wouldn't consider getting my hair cut anywhere else. How many other establishments provided a stand-up comedy performance while you waited to be transformed into an irresistible showpiece!

I walked up the wooden sidewalk to the beauty parlour that sat opposite the high school. As usual the place was hopping. Both chairs were occupied. Norm was snipping away at the back of a head of grey-black hair that belonged to Reverend Tanner. Tom was flitting around the caped form of a pudgy middle-aged woman, plucking curlers from tightly wound, vibrantly blonde hair and tossing them into a plastic tray.

"Oh, look who's here for his overhaul!" Tom chimed. "What's the matter, Doc, did the cows tell you that you were too ugly to put your arm up their arses? You look like a bloody hippie."

I sidled into the room without responding. The last thing Tom needed was encouragement. While he ranted, I sorted through the selection of magazines and periodicals on the rack. I chose a copy of the *National Enquirer* with Liz Taylor on the cover. She was getting divorced again.

"One of us will try and make you look human as soon as we're done. Norm's just about finished with Father Divine. Although I've got a bigger challenge." Tom gestured toward the client in his chair. He sighed, stood back, and shook his head. "I have to make this old broad look sexy…I'll be here all day."

The woman—I recognized her as a teller from the Bank of Commerce—burst into laughter. I was never able to figure how Tom could get away with the comments he made. Anyone else would have been drawn and quartered long ago.

The moment my butt hit the waiting room chair, Belinda the poodle trotted over and hopped onto my knee. The dog was immaculately groomed with a puff at the tip of her tail and another on the top of her head. The undisputed queen of the establishment, she had the run of the place and her greatest hardship was deciding whose lap to occupy. Today Belinda's hair was her natural apricot colour. The last time I saw her, she had been dyed green to help St. Patrick celebrate his birthday.

"You may as well give up on Dr. Dave, Belinda," Norm hollered across the room. "Every other bitch in town is chasing him, too."

"A shame to waste a good-looking guy like you on women," Tom jibed.

I held the *Enquirer* in front of my face as the boys rattled on. I had long ago discovered that the best way to avoid feeding the fire was to keep my mouth shut. In fact, it didn't take long for Tom to give up on me and start chattering away at Reverend Tanner about how they were going to drag Mother Divine on a gambling trip. The good reverend sat there stoically listening to how the boys would take his wife to Vegas and introduce her to Satan.

Norm flicked the cape from the reverend's shoulders. "Okay, you old fart, time to get out there and save some more souls."

The reverend stood and brushed a clump of hair from his pant leg. "Well, thank you for the trim, boys." He paid Norm, and the till chimed as he headed for the door.

Tom fired one more parting volley. "At least you know that when Mother Divine travels with us, she's perfectly safe."

Norm turned to me. "Okay! Let's see what you smell like today."

He directed me to a chair in front of the wash sink. The moment I settled, Tom slipped over and stuck his nose into my collar. He rolled his eyes and made an impish face. "Mmm, he smells hot."

"What do you mean?" Norm queried. "No cows, no pigs?"

"I was a small animal vet all day," I countered.

"Cripes," Tom feigned. "The last time you were in, you'd just come from a dairy barn. You had shit all over your collar and I damn near had to shear your locks with a clothespin on my nose."

Norm wrapped a plastic cloak around my neck and doused my hair with a flow of warm water. I lay there enjoying the feeling of his fingertips massaging my scalp. I could get used to being spoiled.

"It's not fair," Tom whined. "You get to work on all the good-looking guys, and I have to perform magic turning all these old boots into ruby slippers."

Tom ran his hands through his client's hair, then covered it with a plastic cap and stuck her under the dryer. He paused, glanced around the room, and lit up a cigarette. He took a deep drag and exhaled it with an exaggerated groan. Grabbing a broom, he swept up the reverend's hair and scooped it into the waste bin.

"Oh, my God," he said suddenly, parking his cigarette in an ashtray, "I forgot Gertrude again."

Grabbing his hand-held mirror, Tom headed directly for the corner where a slight white-haired lady slumped beneath a dryer.

73

He held the glass under her nose and feigned keen interest.

"Damn, she's still with us. Looks like I'll have to comb her out." He gently shook her arm. "Gert! Gert! Wake up, sweetie! Time to get you combed out, dear."

The woman stirred and Tom helped her to her feet. Together they tottered to his chair.

"That's a girl, Gert. Did you have a good sleep, dearie?"

The poor woman moved as if still in a daze. Yawning, she looked vacantly around her.

"Last week," Tom said, "we were all locked up and I was sweeping the floor after supper. I couldn't believe it—just about had a kitten when I saw poor old Gert still sitting there. She'd slept through the entire afternoon."

I laughed. "What did you do?"

"I gassed her with hairspray and called her a cab."

Norm wrapped a towel around my head and escorted me to his chair. "Well, at least she kept her teeth in today," he commented.

Tom laughed. "A couple months ago I went to check how dry she was, and there were her dentures sitting on her boobs. I didn't know what to do—I didn't want to embarrass her. So I picked them up and tried stuffing them back in. She kept getting her tongue in the way, and I finally had to wake her up."

Norm stood back and surveyed my profile. "Oh God, Dave, you have to let me at those sideburns. If they get any longer, you'll look like Abe Lincoln."

"Don't you think you should cut him short today, Norm?" Tom suggested. "Long hair is out and it's time he stopped looking like one of the Grateful Dead."

Tom leafed through a magazine and showed me the picture of a handsome male model with short-cropped hair. He raised his eyebrows. "Isn't he a hottie? Of course, it would take more than a haircut to make you look like him."

I shook my head and turned to Norm. "Just a trim. I had my

fill of short haircuts when I was a kid. My old man would hack away with a pair of shears that pulled out as much hair as they clipped."

"I remember those," Tom announced. "My mother always used a pair on us, too."

"And I have this bump across the back of my head that Dad refused to hide." I reflexively reached around to feel the indentation. "Man, I hated that..."

Norm lit a cigarette and took a drag. "Trust me," he said somewhat menacingly.

I smiled a little uncomfortably. Setting his cigarette in the ashtray on his carousel, Norm brought his scissors to my hair.

"Just not...not too, too much," I said, trying for diplomacy.

I watched the cigarette smoke curl toward the ceiling, then turned my eyes back to the mirror as Norm made a few quick, efficient snip-snips. For the first time in a long time, my ear was partially exposed.

Norm stopped to look at me, assessing my reaction. Once he realized I wasn't going to throttle him, he returned to his dodge-and-parry scissor technique. In lightning speed I was done. It wasn't exactly a crewcut, but it was shorter than I was used to.

"Well, your highness?" Norm positioned a mirror at arm's length. "What do you think?"

"It looks all right," I said.

"All right! I work my fingers to the bloody bone to try and please you, and you say it looks *all right?*"

I went to stand up, but Tom pushed me back in the seat. "Wait. Wait." He grabbed a bottle from under the counter and sprinkled my hair and the back of my neck with a clear pink solution.

"Oh, my God!" I gagged. "What is that?"

"Rosewater," Tom chirped with a smile. "It'll make you smell pretty for all your four-legged friends."

"Smell pretty, hell!" I gasped, still trying to catch my breath. "More likely cause a stampede."

75

When I returned to the office, Doris chimed, "Well, that looks better. I swear I can even see your ears." She sniffed at the air. "Mmm…don't you smell pretty!"

Shirley Douthwright smiled at me from where she sat on a bench in the waiting room, a large black and white cat on her lap. Shirley was a waitress at the Depot Restaurant.

"Hi, Shirley," I said, doing my best to ignore Doris. "I was just at Manell's House of Beauty."

Shirley nodded. "So I gather. Always an experience, huh?"

Doris wasn't going to be muscled out of the conversation so easily. "I'll say it's an experience! I don't know how anyone takes the boys' abuse, but at least Tom gets this guy looking halfway human. And *that's* no mean feat."

Doris jerked her thumb at me, then handed over Shirley's admission card. "Moose is here for his vaccinations."

I tried not to let Doris see me smile at her own loving abuse as I headed to the back room to get my smock. At least I couldn't smell rosewater anymore—the sickly sweet scent had pretty much burned out my olfactory bulb. I fumbled with the ties of the smock as I approached the examining table. Shirley carried her big cat in her arms.

"So how's Moose been, Shirley?"

The petite blonde carefully settled her cat on the table. She ran her hand the length of his body and deposited the loose hair in the wastebasket.

"You know, there's more to him than meets the eye."

I looked at the cat expectantly, thinking that I was about to hear a story about Moose's antics. Every client was certain theirs was the smartest, most talented, and, yes, even the most psychic pet in the valley. But, in fact, Shirley wasn't talking about Moose at all.

"In June I got a call that my mother died. I decided to fly home for the funeral even though it would cost me money I didn't have, 'cause of the divorce and everything…"

She paused a moment and focused on scraping a bit of caked-on dirt from the tip of the cat's ear.

"Anyway, I called up Tom for an appointment to get my hair done before leaving town. He said, 'There's no way, Shirley. I'm up to my ass in teeny-boppers—tonight's grad night.' But I guess he could tell by the sound of my voice that something was wrong. When he found out why I wanted the appointment, he said, 'Be here at twelve-thirty...' You know, he did my hair and made other people wait. When I tried to pay him..."

She paused and tears glistened in her eyes. "He took me aside at the back of the shop and told me that there was no charge... then asked if I needed money for my trip. I didn't know what to say. I'm fifty-five years old and no one had ever given me a free hairdo before."

"That's our Tom," chimed Doris from the doorway

That's our Tom, indeed, I thought.

The door had barely closed behind Shirley and Moose when Doris turned and levelled her gaze at me.

"Your next appointment is at the Hurfords," she said.

From the look on her face, I knew I didn't want to hear the rest. She took a deep breath before she continued. "Herb called just before you got back...said to make sure you have lots of fluids for the IV."

A wave of fatigue washed over me. Doris's news was something I hoped I wouldn't hear, but somewhere in the back of my mind, deep down, I knew it was just a matter of time. I steeled myself and took a look at the day page on Doris's desk. It read: *Tsolum Farms—mastitis cow—manure-like water—hardly able to stand. Best cow on the farm—Herb will do anything to save her.* Doris watched me carefully.

"Damn...I was hoping we had seen the last of them."

Four days ago the vaccine that Jeremy Greenfield had prepared arrived from the provincial lab. After trying the concoction on a couple of guinea-pig cows, we had waited two days and watched for adverse reactions. When nothing seemed unusual with them, we inoculated the entire herd.

Doris nodded her head in sympathy. "They know you're doing your best, Dave."

A welcome vote of confidence, but clearly my best had not been good enough. The day we vaccinated the cows, almost half the milk was going down the drain, and Herb was scared spitless because a hired hand may have milked a treated cow too soon. It would be a disaster if he got caught shipping milk containing antibiotic residues.

Herb met me at the milk-house door. He looked exhausted.

"Thanks for coming, Dave." Grabbing a five-gallon bucket, he began filling it with water. For a brief moment he paused to sniff at the air, unsure where the unusual, sickly sweet smell was coming from. Out of politeness, he said nothing, but I could see the confusion pass over his face. I must still smell to high heaven of Tom's magic potion.

"Where are the boys?" I asked, surprised to see him out here—it was usually Danny or David who helped with the cows.

Herb sighed. "They don't want anything to do with her," he said with a hint of disgust. "Danny wanted to get the gun and shoot her. I know he's right, but I have to try—122 is the best cow on the farm—a purebred from my foundation herd back on the Island. I just can't give up on her without a struggle."

He turned off the hose, picked up the bucket, and limped off into the milk house. I had never seen him in so much discomfort before. He had arthritic knees, but prided himself on never letting that slow him down. I guess there's something about hard times that brings out aches and pains. We arrived at the plywood door to the calving pen.

"She's worse now than she was when I called. You don't think it could have been that damned vaccine, do you?"

I shook my head. "The bug would have been killed with formaldehyde as part of the process. I'm afraid that we just didn't have enough time to develop immunity for her—it hasn't even been two days."

"Both back teats were already blue when I looked at her an hour ago…She just delivered last night. Danny pre-milked her and treated her quarters preventively, but it didn't seem to do a bit of good. He swears her milk was still clean last night. This morning we saw a trace on the mastitis test, so we ran her back in at lunch just to be sure…"

Herb set down his bucket and fumbled with a twine that held the door closed. It swung open to reveal a huge Holstein cow stretched out on her side.

"I just can't understand it, Dave. We dug this pen down to new dirt and hauled in sand. How could she have caught something from here?" He stared at me intently. "Where are they getting this damned bug?" He looked at the cow, shook his head in disgust. "And why 122?" he muttered.

Why 122? I asked myself Herb's question again. Why were some cows more susceptible than others? Why hadn't we seen a heifer affected? Why were only newly calved cows susceptible? It had to be some type of environmental mastitis.

From deep in her throat, #122 released a low groan. Lifting her head for a moment, she let it fall back to the straw-covered ground with a sickening thud. She took a few rapid breaths and groaned again. Her eyes were sunken, her muzzle crusted with straw.

I lifted a manure-sodden tail and slipped a thermometer into her rectum. Immediately, it was ejected along with a stream of dirty brown water. I gingerly lifted her tail and poked around in the muck with a stick. Retrieving the thermometer, I replaced it.

I knelt beside the cow and palpated her udder. The two back quarters were as cold as ice, and both teats were the colour of ripe plums. The front quarters were as hard as rock as well. I squirted material from the back quarters. Only clear purple water came out—not a hint of anything that could be considered milk. I squirted fluid from the front quarters—both were tinged with blood, but still identifiable as milk. I reached for the thermometer. Her temperature was 37.8—a degree below normal.

"She looks rough, Herb. There's no way those hindquarters will ever produce milk again." I had trouble looking in the man's direction.

"My best cow. I wanted a heifer from her in the worst way, Dave. This time she had a bull."

"We can pump some fluids into her and start an IV, but we haven't done too well with that in the past. This bug is obviously putting out a serious toxin that the animal is absorbing."

"Is there something else we can do? Anything just to get another chance at a heifer—even if I never get another drop of milk from her."

"Well…" I went through the medical scenarios in my head, "when we're dealing with gangrene in other organs and other species, we would definitely consider amputation. The udder is the main source of the poison right now, and removing it could well make a difference…Given that the milk is not your priority."

"You mean cut off her entire bag?"

I nodded.

"Have you ever done that?"

"I've amputated quarters before, but never an entire udder."

I was suggesting a radical solution, and Herb knew it. The surgery was almost unthinkable—removing such a massive part of the cow's body. I'd never seen a study of how much blood actually passes through the udder of a Holstein cow during the first week of her lactation, but I wouldn't be surprised if it wasn't one-third of her entire output. What a daunting thought. Besides that, I had never heard of anyone preserving a dairy cow without an udder.

What else was there? Fluids and antibiotic treatment had failed every other cow.

Herb scratched his head. "If you're willing to try…"

"Yeah. I am." The fact was, I hated quitting and I couldn't stand the thought that this disease would take another animal out from under me. I wanted to beat it just as much as my client did.

Herb nodded. "Just tell me what you need."

We were going to do this thing.

"We better get some fluids into her—start an intravenous right now and pump some in before we leave her."

I carried my surgical supplies from the car and made a second trip for ropes and a five-gallon container of intravenous fluids. I shaved the cow's tail end and administered thirty millilitres of lidocaine as an epidural. Once her hind legs were paralyzed, we struggled to roll the cow onto her back. I secured ropes to each of her legs.

Hanging the five gallon carboy of fluids from a rafter above us, I adjusted the plastic coils of the IV line so they would be out of the way. Herb held his hand at the base of the cow's neck to build pressure on the jugular vein while I drove a three-inch catheter into the vessel. Blood gushed forth and I removed the metal stylus. I hooked on the intravenous line and watched as fluids flowed in a steady stream through the drip chamber.

"Could you hold this for me, Herb?"

Leaning toward me, my assistant grasped the rubber tubing. I stepped away quickly, retrieved a needle from my cold sterilization tray, and threaded it with suture material. Driving it through the skin of the cow's neck, I tied the material around the catheter.

As I shaved the hair from the underbelly, I was barraged by a steady stream of negative self-talk. *Who would ever consider a fool thing like this? What good's a cow without an udder, anyway? What happens to an impaired circulatory system when you tie off major vessels and remove a hundred pounds of tissue from a cow's body?*

I shook my head and continued clipping around the huge milk veins on the cow's ventral abdomen. I had sutured a hole in one before and had tremendous respect for the amount of blood that could gush in a matter of seconds from a vessel the size of a garden hose.

"Better get another bucket of water for me to scrub in," I said as I slopped the reddish-brown soap over the periphery of the udder and began washing it.

By the time I had the drapes positioned and installed a blade on the scalpel handle, I was ready to get started. I began my incision twelve inches in front of the udder and angled sideways, toward the milk vein. I was dismayed by the blood that oozed from the wound margins. It was the same purple-red hue as the necrotic teats on the cow's udder—the toxins were hard at work.

I continued the incision, first down one side of the udder then the other, staying as high on the gland as possible in order to have enough skin left to close the defect. I dissected around both milk veins, which were surprisingly flat and difficult to see. It must have had something to do with her lying on her back, because when she was upright, they were more than an inch across. I ligated the right side, carefully anchoring the suture to the underlying tissue. Cranking down hard on the synthetic, stringlike suture material, I threw on several more knots. If this stitch were to fail, the cow would pump her entire blood volume on the ground within minutes.

I placed a second suture on the udder side and cut between the two. I repeated the procedure on the other side, and then began lifting and separating the huge gland from the gleaming white surface of the cow's underbelly. I trimmed away at the tissue of the suspensory apparatus with my scissors, cutting through the tough gristly material that held the udder tight to the cow's body.

A rivulet of sweat trickled across my forehead. I backed away from the cow and shook myself to dislodge the drops somewhere other than my surgery site.

Herb watched me work with a look of solemn resignation. What an ordeal this had to be for him. Watching me remove an udder from his best cow had to be similar to a coach watching surgeons remove a leg from his star quarterback. Neither patient would ever again do what they had been born to do.

I struggled to lift the forward portion of the udder enough to get a clear view of the site. My left arm trembled from the exertion, while my right snipped onwards.

"I'm going to need assistance, Herb. If you scrub up, I'll get you to hold the gland up so I can see what I'm doing."

It was at this point that I found myself fighting to hide my steadily increasing anxiety from my client. Any large animal vet was familiar with the large blood vessels that *drained* the udder area—these vessels were huge and close to the surface. The ones that we often saw damaged by barbed wire or manure scrapers in the barn—they required our attention frequently enough to be considered routine. But the arteries that *supplied* the udder were another matter entirely. Though somewhat smaller, they were totally buried from sight. Many animal anatomy books barely touched on them, presumably because a vet would seldom have any need to operate so deeply into the cow's innards. I was dealing with an unusual circumstance, knowing full well that an accidental cut to a critical supply vessel would spell an immediate bath in blood and a quick end to 122's life.

Herb finished scrubbing before he stepped forward to take the weight of the cow's udder. As he hefted, I crammed my hand deep beneath the gland in search of a pulsating vessel, so that I could avoid severing it. I cut away more of the gristly material, and Herb leaned back until the mammary gland was almost upside down.

"Hold it steady."

I worked away at the connective tissue on the left side until I located the vessel. The huge artery throbbing beneath my fingers pulsated with each contraction of the heart. I passed a needle around it and cranked hard on the ends of the suture material. It wouldn't do for a ligature on this vessel to let go. I tied off another massive vein, then cut through more material. Severing the skin at the back of the udder, I worked my way to the right.

We were almost finished—just one more set of vessels to tie off and the udder would be excised.

There was a flurry of movement. I felt a sharp pain in the centre of my back as 122's front leg deflected off my spine. Struggling frantically, the cow pumped her front legs back and forth against the restraints. Herb looked apprehensive as he steadfastly held his position.

The legs went limp and I continued my dissection. It was the look on Herb's face that brought me up short. I turned and stared at the cow's chest.

She had stopped breathing—122 was dead.

Herb looked silently at the floor as we finished our beer. At first he had tried to cover his disappointment, but I knew just how hard it had hit him.

A good vet is part doctor, part therapist, and when a man loses a prize like 122, the vet's medical skills take a back seat to his or her ability to counsel. But what more could I say? I'd failed him. The bug was beating me. It was time for me to crawl away, preferably under a nice big rock. I stood to leave and Herb stood, too.

"I know you feel bad, Dave."

I nodded. "I really tried. I just keep wondering if there was something I could've done differently—"

Herb raised his hands to stop me there. He smiled.

"I never saw a vet try so hard. I don't think there's anything else you could do…Well, maybe just one thing."

My heart skipped a beat. What other weaknesses had I revealed?

"What's that?" I asked, waiting for his wisdom.

"Just…don't wear that godawful perfume out here again …You're damn near choking me to death."

Trick-or-Treat

"Oh man, Dave, I think I'm gonna be sick!"

David Hurford screwed up his face as gallons of putrid-smelling fluid spewed forth from the cow's back end. I jumped to the side, twisting my long body in a vain attempt to avoid the blood-tinged torrent. Swallowing reflexively, I dolefully glanced downward. The right leg of my coveralls was soaked. A fine layer of hair clung to the cotton fabric like an art deco design. An occasional unidentifiable gob or string of organic matter augmented the pattern. I wiggled my toes as the warm sensation slowly penetrated and crept farther and farther downward. Was my boot full yet? Too soon to tell.

"Why didn't she push if she's been ready to calf for so long?" The handsome young dairyman maintained a hold on the cow's tail. He plugged his nose with his free hand and looked away from me in disgust. "The only reason I even noticed her was that bit of crap on her tail. Then I got close and got a whiff—I could tell right away something was wrong."

"The calf was coming backwards," I wheezed, "and because nothing entered the pelvis but the tail, she could see no reason to push." I reached forward through the partially closed cervix to try and get a better feel for the situation.

"I wish Danny were here," David gasped. "He's got a stronger stomach than I have."

I dragged in another stilted breath as the stench settled like smog over the mucous membranes of my nasal cavity. What a fine way to end a day—what a fine way to celebrate Halloween!

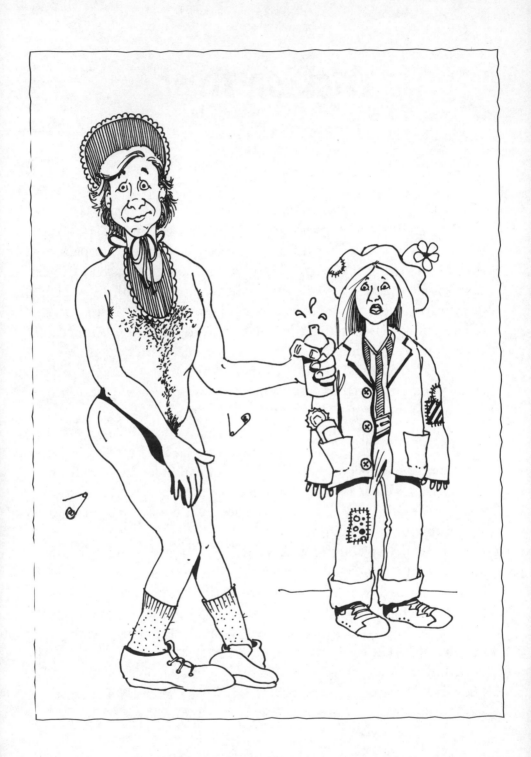

"Can you do anything with her?" David's face was ashen. Although he still held onto the cow's tail, he was standing about as far from me as his arm would allow.

"It's a tough call." I adjusted my plastic sleeve, then pressed forward into the heifer to the full extent of my reach. "The cervix isn't fully open anymore…We get reefing around too much and we could tear her."

"Can you do a Caesarian on a critter like her?" David asked half-heartedly.

"We could," I mused, "but you can see how rotten this calf is. It's probably been dead in her for ages. It's in the condition I'd picture a corpse after three days in the hot sun. If some of this crap gets into her abdomen, we can kiss her goodbye."

"Wouldn't you know it?" David groaned. "We needed her milk in the worst way…After all the trouble over this darned mastitis, we're not even close to filling our quota. We'd have normally had her up here a couple of weeks ago where we could watch her closer—but you told us to calve them out on the dike where the ground was clean."

I nodded glumly. I had told them to allow as many cows as possible to deliver on pasture—away from ground that could be contaminated. This mastitis situation was threatening to be the end of me as well as the Hurfords.

I had performed post-mortem exams on six cows so far. Although all of them died before the use of the bacterin, that didn't mean things were any better. Far from it. As a matter of fact, many animals got frightfully ill in spite of vaccination, and the sick pens were now plugged with cows, some wandering around with great hunks of udder sloughing from their body. In some ways, they were more of a liability alive than if they had died.

But in early October there had been a bright spot—hell no, a breakthrough. Because none of the specialists I talked to had heard of *Bacillus cereus* as a cause of mastitis, I contacted the librarian at the Western College of Veterinary Medicine in

Saskatoon and asked him to do a literature search for me.

He apologized when he came back with only two references—one published in the *Australian Veterinary Journal* describing a farmer who had done his own teat surgery and accidentally introduced the bug, and the other, a paper from the *Journal of the American Veterinary Association*. That was the one that knocked my socks off. It described an outbreak in cows that occurred during a trial when a new mastitis preparation was being developed for release in the American market. I flushed with horror as I read—the antibiotic implicated in that outbreak was the exact same one we were using as our main drug in the dry-cow mastitis program on Tsolum Farms. They were still going through cases of the product per week. Had following my recommendations gotten one of my best clients into all this misery?

That very night I packaged up bottles of the suspect product from my own shelf and shipped them off. One went to the provincial veterinary lab, one to Food and Drug in Ottawa, and one to Dr. Ward in the bacteriology department at the Western College of Veterinary Medicine. Three days ago, Dr. Ward had called to tell me that he had grown *Bacillus cereus* from the product.

How could that be? How could an antibiotic that was prepared under sterile conditions—one that was designed to kill bacteria—possibly harbour one?

I cringed as I remembered relating the news to Herb. He was silent for the longest time, then ranted about how a company could be allowed to put out a product that caused disease. All *he* was trying to do was prevent one. I revisited the shame I felt as I hung my head, feeling that I deserved every bit of his wrath. After all, I was as complicit as I could be. Not only had I recommended the product, I had sold it to him.

I sighed and forced myself to get back to the job at hand. Pulling the plastic glove tight to my armpit, I stretched as far forward as I could reach. This calf was disgusting—bloated beyond recognition. Fluid and gas bubbled beneath its skin; hair peeled away from it like mould from the surface of a rotting plum. I withdrew just as the heifer pushed. Another gallon of watery fluid mixed with clumps of hair spurted from her vagina. David shot me a look of despair.

I cringed and drew in a breath. The stench was beyond comprehension. "I'm going to try and take this out through the back end. You get a couple more buckets of water while I get the embryotome."

David happily released the heifer's tail and disappeared in the direction of the milk house. As I retrieved my equipment from my car, I kept a close eye on the house—I hated the prospect of running into Herb today. The problem with this heifer was bad enough; the last thing I needed was for him to corner me and start fuming about the ongoing mastitis fiasco. The entire family was demoralized, so much so that Danny had taken a few days off and escaped to the Coast. It was the first time since I'd started working in the valley that I had known him to leave the farm for more than a few hours at a time.

I struggled to manipulate a calving handle in front of the hind leg of the fetus. With the partially closed cervix and the distension of the corpse, room to maneuver was non-existent. Abandoning the instrument as far forward as I could poke it, I withdrew, passed my hand between the calf's legs, and searched for the metal D of the calving hook again. Finally grasping it, I pulled the handle with the wire attached back out the vagina.

"How in the world do you expect to cut anything with that stuff?" David looked askance at the woven wire that for all the world resembled something used for hanging picture frames.

I passed a three-foot needle through the embryotome, a long, tubular, stainless-steel apparatus that would protect the vaginal wall from the abrasion of the wire. "You'll soon see." I pulled the wire out the far end, screwed a handle to each end of the cable, and motioned for David to start sawing. "Just pull with one, then the other—no jerks—just long, even strokes." I reached into the vagina again. Wedging the head of the instrument on the opposite side of the tail, I nodded for my helper to proceed.

He leaned back on one handle, then the other and maintained pressure on the wire, working steadily back and forth. For three or four minutes, his pulls met with constant resistance, and the air resonated with a low-pitched grinding sound. Slowly, the wires increased in length.

Suddenly, there was the sound of metal abrading metal, and the entire apparatus pulled from the womb. I passed the bloody instrument to David and worked my hand back into the uterus. I probed gingerly over a jagged structure. The wire had severed the calf's hind leg from its body by passing through the centre of the hip. I felt for the tail, cushioned the sharp protuberance of the pelvic bones with my hand, and gradually manipulated the piece through the heifer's birth canal.

David took a deep breath and looked away as I withdrew the inflated body part and tossed it on the ground behind me. "Oh man, that's gross," he groaned.

I rinsed gobs of clinging hair from my sleeve and unhooked the handle from the wire. Removing one end from the embryotome, I maneuvered back into the heifer. How disgusting to think of removing this fetus one piece at a time. But what choice did we have? I passed the wire around the back of the calf's bloated abdomen, making sure to stay well ahead of its pelvis. Threading the embryotome again, I handed the apparatus to David and nodded. He pulled hesitantly on first one handle, then the other until his motions gathered momentum and became more fluid.

I watched his expression as he heaved back and forth. Progress seemed slower this time, and beads of sweat soon popped out on his forehead. As he raised his hand to mop his brow, he noticed the blood and hair clinging to his fingers. He stopped in disgust, stared at me in desperation, then leaned back to start sawing with renewed vigour.

With my arm buried deep in the heifer's uterus, I watched my friend's struggle. Although at this point in the procedure, I was little more than an observer, I had no illusions that it would remain that way. Holding the instrument firmly to the calf's spine, I focused on the vibration of the wire as it grumbled its way through rotten flesh.

"Has it quit cutting?" David gasped after a period of prolonged exertion. "I'm about done in."

As if in answer to his question, metal ground upon metal, and the apparatus lunged in his direction. He clutched the handle before the tool hit the ground and stumbled toward a bucket of water to clean himself. I cautiously felt my way around the perimeter of the newly severed piece of calf. Pushing forward on the pelvis, I jammed it beneath the abdomen of the remaining torso and followed the leg to the hock. I flexed it, grasped the hoof, and applied steady traction. The leg straightened; I brought the foot out through the vaginal lips.

David's disgust intensified when the horny covering of the hoof peeled free to plop on the ground, and the small pink bones pointed toward the sky. Slipping a chain around the fetlock, I looked expectantly in his direction.

"Pass me one of those hooks, will you?" I secured the handle to the chain and extended it to my helper, then squirted Bridine soap in my cupped hand and coated the lining of the vagina in an attempt to lubricate it. The mucous that was normally present at a birthing had been broken down by putrefaction, and the membranes of the vagina felt rough and dry. "Lean back gently...slow, steady tension."

I kept my hand jammed over the jagged edge of the pelvis, moving with it as David coaxed the hind leg from the womb. He shook his head as it landed with a splat on the toe of his boot. Soaping my sleeve again, I drove my hand into the now exposed abdomen of the calf and pulled forth yard after yard of bowel.

"My God!" David exclaimed at the grey-blue mound building at my feet. "You're worse than a dog on a gut heap."

He didn't look when the greyish mass representing the liver and diaphragm hit the dirt. He cringed at the deep tearing sound that vibrated through the heifer when my fingers grasped the decaying flesh of the heart and lungs and wrenched it from its mooring. It wasn't until I grabbed a pair of ribs and started reefing that he had to leave.

"I need some air," he gasped.

When I withdrew my hand, I was trembling from exertion. Dropping the pale red shards of bone onto the growing heap of debris, I opened and closed my aching fingers. The plastic sleeve that had been offering a psychological barrier between this rotting mass and my flesh was riddled with holes. Watery pink fluid sloshed back and forth in the fingers, and my skin stuck suspiciously to the plastic. I pulled the glove off and raised my elbow to my nose. I'd be smelling this for a week.

I was convinced that removal of the supporting structure of the ribs and sternum would permit the remainder of the carcass to pass intact. Soaping my arms, I probed the vagina and resumed my attack—two ribs from one side, two from the other, a handful from the sternum. How many ribs were there, anyway? Drifting back to the anatomy lab at veterinary college, I pictured Aaron Horowitz at my elbow grilling me. His intense blue eyes bored into me; his forehead was etched in its perpetual frown. Were there twelve more? Fourteen? Damned if I could remember. By the time I had torn away the last bone, I was exhausted. I had lost count of how many ribs I had pulled out, and still had not the faintest idea how many I had started with.

David returned as I slipped a chain over the remains of the calf's spine and made certain that it had a good bite. I nodded for him to start pulling and held my arm in place until it was obvious that the shoulders of the fetus could squeeze through the cervix. Then I grabbed a handle and began straining along with him.

Progress was aggravated by a total lack of mucous and by the fact that we were working against the grain of the hair. The shoulders were just emerging when the heifer emitted a plaintive bawl and flopped onto her side. David and I staggered backwards as the bloated remnants of the corpse spewed onto the ground. The "calf" was delivered.

It was after seven by the time I got back to the office. David was aware of how distressed I was with the antibiotic issues and had kindly only mentioned it in passing. Lug was at the door to greet me. Jamming his nose into my right boot, he snuffled and carried on as if I had a treat hidden there for him.

Doris was long gone. A pile of Halloween toffee sporting traditional orange and black wrappers sat on the daybook. A note from my faithful sidekick lay under them. *Happy Halloween!* it read. I meticulously unwrapped one of the packets, getting the treat to my mouth without its touching my odiferous fingers.

Munching on the candy, I followed my exuberant pet up the stairs. Doris and I had been joking this morning about trick-or-treating, and even though she'd left me a treat, I knew she wasn't above concocting a trick. It was with a sense of disappointment that I got as far as the tub without discovering some sort of booby trap...Surely there should be more to Halloween than this.

I closed my eyes and submerged my head in the water. Soap bubbles crackled and popped as they burst at my temples. I came up for air and attacked my arms with the bar of soap. The smell of that rotten calf continued to follow me like a shadow. Although I knew from experience that only time would allow it to fade, I was determined to do something to dull it.

I grabbed the bottle of lemon juice from the side of the tub and squirted the cold solution down the length of my arm. The first treatment certainly didn't cut the mustard, but maybe one more application would help. Rubbing it in, I added an extra dab to the armpit. After rinsing, I took another whiff. The wretched smell lived on. Granted, there were overtones of Irish Spring soap and Colgate toothpaste, but it was there.

I climbed from the tub and wandered into the kitchen, still rubbing my back with a towel. I should have gone to bed for a good night's sleep, but for some reason I felt restless. Grabbing the armload of clean laundry Doris had left on the table, I headed into the bedroom. That woman never ceased to amaze me. It had been so busy today—I wouldn't have thought she'd have time for laundry, yet here everything was, neatly folded for me to put away. I stuffed my underwear into the top drawer of the dresser, then grabbed a pair of jeans, and parked them on a shelf in the closet.

I tossed a pair of crisply folded white sheets onto the bed, picked up the top one, and caressed it dreamily. I drifted back in memory. I had unearthed an old Japanese-orange box in the closet when I was looking for my college transcripts a couple of days ago. Now I rummaged through it and picked out a baby bottle with a big rubber nipple, a frilly blue bonnet, and a plastic bib. Tipping the remaining contents onto the bed, I spread out the collection of odds and ends. After I set aside an assortment of old greeting cards, note pads, and half-used pencils, I found what I was looking for—two big blue safety pins.

I laughed out loud as I recalled the night that Mrs. Gartner had given me this stuff. It was during a particularly cold stretch in February 1971—two years before my graduation. Why the founding students at Western College had established a tradition of putting on a masquerade party in the middle of the winter was beyond me—but there it was, advertised as the "third annual."

Ron Zdriluk and Jim Carnie had been pestering me for weeks about hitting the books too hard. It was only after their constant harangue that I decided to ask Pat Nelson, a home economics major staying at the same boarding house as I was, if she wanted to go to the ball. I warned her that the animals who attended the vet college were wilder than the ones they worked on, but she assured me she was a stalwart farm girl and was up to it. We were to ride to the party together with the Carnies and Zdriluks.

I had given little thought to what I would wear to the function until that final day. Pat had asked me repeatedly if I had decided on a costume yet. She was obviously hoping to come up with some idea for herself. I was too concerned about what Dr. Gupta would ask on the pharmacology quiz to give too much thought to such triviality.

It was after five that Friday when I finished cleaning up from the physiology lab and headed to the locker room. I rushed through the door and slammed on the brakes. My God! What were these two strange women doing in our change room? At that moment the buxom, squarely built woman with the long black hair turned to face me. Shoving her hand down the front of her gold mini-dress, she fished out a huge grapefruit.

"Man, Carnie, can't I use lemons? These are too big."

"Zdriluk?" I stared in disbelief at the bizarre couple. The blonde in the white chiffon dress turned and rubbed her hand on my chest.

"Hello there, big fella."

I was peering into the mischievous blue eyes of my classmate. "My God, Carnie, you and big Z are downright frightening in those getups."

"What're you wearing?" Zdriluk demanded, replacing the grapefruit and staring at his sagging breast with a measure of disgust.

I shrugged my shoulders. "I don't have a costume yet."

"Well, you better decide pretty quickly," Carnie asserted. "'Cause you can't go to the party without a costume. We'll be picking you up at quarter to eight."

"Well, how about you give me a dress, too?"

"Sorry, man…How many dresses do ya think I own? The wife's got me on a budget."

Had I left this too late? Maybe I should call Pat and tell her to forget about tonight—we'd just stay home.

I threw on my scarf, zipped up my coat, and made a beeline for the exit. I burst out the door into air so cold that I had to work my eyes to keep my lids from freezing shut—there'd be no time for dawdling tonight. I yanked my toque from my pocket and pulled it down over my ears. I usually hated anything on my head, but there was something about thirty-below weather that had given me an appreciation for wool.

I got home and thrashed about my room looking for anything that could be turned into a costume. But I was living a pretty stark existence in Saskatoon, with only a few changes of clothing. This was not going to be easy. It was the curtains that got me thinking. I kept looking at their ugly green floral pattern and wondering what I could do with them…If I sewed them both together, they'd make a skirt, but what would I do for the rest of the outfit?

A toga? Not anywhere near big enough…but the bed sheet might just do it. I pulled off the quilt and tugged at the sheet. It was a single size—white cotton. I draped it over my body, trying to remember how the Romans wore those things, but quickly decided that no respectable republican would be caught dead in a bed sheet.

A ghost. I draped the sheet over my head—it was only long enough to cover me to my waist. I'd be the ghost who wore blue jeans.

I wandered upstairs with sheet in hand and knocked on my landlady's door. She was a practical sort and had raised three children of her own. Surely, she'd have some sort of an idea—maybe she even had a costume she could lend me.

Just over five feet with her heels on, Mrs. Gartner was a sprightly woman in her mid-seventies. She looked at me with a twinkle in her eyes. Biting her lip, she adjusted the comb in her flaming red hair. "Well, my husband Albert was five six—I can't think of anything we have other than our tent that would cover you."

I smiled meekly and started to retreat down the stairs.

"But that sheet of yours might be big enough to make a diaper," she chuckled.

"A diaper?"

She nodded. "You can go as a baby. I dressed my son Fred up as one once."

I blanched. She was just trying to help, after all. Mrs. Gartner took the sheet and quickly folded it on her kitchen table. Tucking it under my behind, she held it in place. "Just a pin here and one here, and you're in business."

"So how did the costume work out for Fred?"

"Not very well," she answered. "He was only seven and refused to leave the house with it on. But he looked so cute!"

I was feeling very much like Fred right then, but if I was going to take Pat to the party tonight, I didn't have much choice.

Mrs. Gartner was sweet enough to painstakingly demonstrate the folding of the diaper with me. How could I refuse? Back in my apartment, I slipped into my bathing suit, then sat on the sheet and pinned up the sides of the bed-sheet diaper. I looked at my reflection in the mirror. The blue of my bathing suit stood out in stark contrast to the white of the diaper. I tucked and pulled, tugged and wrenched. No manner of contortion could hide that insufferable blue.

Stripping down again, I wore the diaper the way any other baby would—bare-arsed. The pins were huge. Taking substantial bites of cloth on either side of my legs, I cinched the diaper tightly. I stood up and hopped from side to side. It felt secure.

I tied on the bonnet and bib Mrs. Gartner had given me. I couldn't suppress a smile. I was rather cute—especially so with strands of my long hair curling up on either side of my temples. Only one thing was missing. Taking the baby bottle to the kitchen, I poured in a few inches of vodka and filled it with orange juice.

My bottle had been refilled a multitude of times, and the hole in the end of the nipple was getting progressively larger. We had created quite a stir when we arrived at the dance, but the moment that stood out most clearly was when Carnie pulled up in front of the liquor store on Circle Drive. I can still see the tall, slender clerk standing there with his mouth agape as we crashed through the door. I guess it wasn't every frigid night he got to serve a half-naked, seven-foot baby and two of the homeliest drag queens that the Prairie provinces had ever produced. "I won't even ask," he said as we went through the till.

The band at the party was exceptional, and their music kept the crowd on its feet throughout most of the evening. Glancing around the hall, I could see that most of the students and faculty had put in an appearance. Pat and I hit it off well and spent most of the evening on the dance floor. She had come dressed as a hobo with a tattered old coat and a big woollen hat pulled over her long blonde locks. Although we might have coordinated our costumes, I doubted that she would have adopted my motif.

The moderator announced a waltz for a spot dance, and everyone crowded onto the floor. Pat snuggled closely with her head on my bare chest. Dean Smith and his wife were dancing next to us. He nodded to me, then nudged his wife and whispered something in her ear. They both turned our way and chuckled. Clutching my baby bottle, I was about as relaxed as I could be. My eyes were closed; we swayed lazily to the music.

It happened without the slightest warning. Before I knew what was going down, Doyle Mulaney and Dale Cochran sneaked up behind me and grabbed the back of my diaper. They both reefed at the same time and safety pins flew. I was standing in the middle of the dance floor clad only in socks, shoes, bib, and bonnet. As if on cue, the band stopped playing and the crowd pulled back. Pat and I were left standing conspicuously in the spotlight. I glanced at the dean and his wife; they were doubled over with laughter.

I fondled the trinkets on the bed for several minutes, thinking back to that memorable night. I smiled, strode to the phone, and dialled Hurfords.

"David, get dressed in something crazy. We're going trick-or-treating."

Saskatoon Revisited

For a man in his twenties, it seemed strange that I gravitated toward older women as assistants and associates. It wasn't as if I planned it that way—it was just the way it worked out.

I never would have hired Doris if it hadn't been at the insistence of my friend, Gordon Veitch. But it didn't take long for the value of her life experience to come into play. She knew the town of Creston inside out, and it was amazing how often that came in handy when we had to collect on an account or track someone down. She always seemed to know that so-and-so's sister worked for Taks or that what's his name's cousin managed the Creston Valley Co-op.

It was during the spring stock-taking for inventory that Doris began to flag. Shirley Shopa had worked earlier in the day, but she had left at five...She was, after all, a wife and mother of two and couldn't be expected to stay late just because it was year-end. I had returned late from a call to the Rogers' farm. Bob's mother, Marg, had prepared supper for us after some routine work at their feedlot. Her husband, Dudley, had died only a few months earlier, and the woman was driving her son nuts with her insistence on helping around the farm.

Doris was dejected at how much remained to be done. She was adamant that she had to finish counting stock before we opened the doors in the morning. I called Marg Rogers to ask if she might want to help. She was there inside half an hour and stayed till the last pill was accounted for.

That had been in March. Now she was the official bookkeeper,

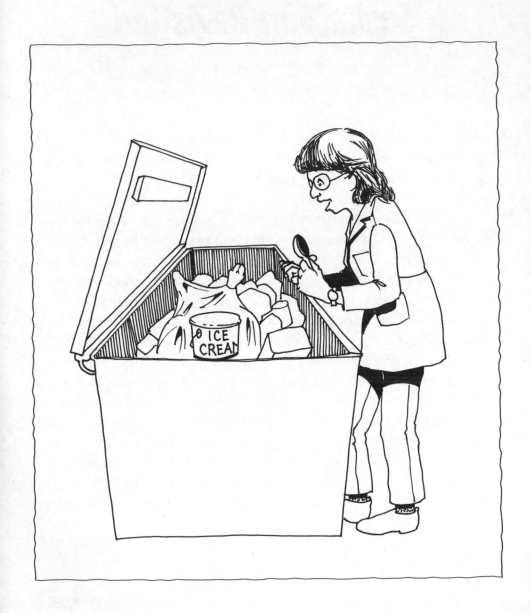

errand runner, and financial manager for Creston Veterinary Clinic. At sixty-seven, she was every bit as full of beans as her teenage granddaughters.

With the accounting and bookkeeping off her plate, Doris was somewhat relieved, but by fall it seemed that all she and I could talk about was how tired we were. It had been a hectic spring, and the long anticipated "summer lull" just didn't happen. In July and August, we had Marcie's help, and Doris managed to avoid a lot of the nighttime call-outs. But now that we were without another hand, the work was beginning to take its toll. Doris and Shirley juggled their spare time trying to maintain sanity, but we all knew they couldn't keep it up.

Doris needed more help, and although I hated to admit it, so did I. All summer long I had been trying to talk myself into hiring a veterinarian to take some of the load. I didn't doubt that there was enough work to keep two of us busy. The challenge would be making sure there was sufficient income to pay another person. I'd just have to learn to charge more to make ends meet.

After hiring two younger women on a trial basis, it became obvious that a career as a veterinary assistant wasn't everyone's cup of tea. The women were bright. They absolutely loved animals, but could not watch a critter endure even a modicum of discomfort. The euthanasia of a road accident victim saw the first promising candidate flee the office in tears. The second was finished when she discovered the tub of ice cream—our afternoon snack—resting on top of a dog corpse in the deep-freeze.

"Margaret Berg would be a good person for here, Dave," Marg Rogers insisted. "I've known her for years, she's not the least bit squeamish, and she knows the meaning of a day's work."

I had always found Mrs. Berg a pleasant woman to be around, and she certainly did seem to be the practical sort. Although I didn't know her well, I'd been to her farm recently to treat her Jersey cow for milk fever. She had insisted that I was looking thin and invited me in for breakfast. A husky farm-girl type, she knew how to throw around a sixty-pound bale of hay. It made me think that she would have no trouble assisting with the animals.

"I'm going over to Nelson to visit Jean next weekend," Doris piped, "so you better get someone before then. Shirley and Alex will be at a calf sale in Alberta."

"How do you know she'd even want a job?"

"She just finished a business course in Nelson," Marg said. "She told me the other day at the West Creston hall meeting that she put her applications in at the Co-op and Websters."

"Give her a try, Dave!" Doris hollered from the surgery. "My kids will soon forget what I look like."

"All right, call her up and see if she can come in tomorrow."

Finding an assistant for the office was proving to be a big enough undertaking. Hiring a second veterinarian for the practice was even more worrisome. I loved the thought of having another person to consult with and challenge my thinking, and I was willing to admit how much I missed Marcie since her departure. Although I hadn't discussed it with anyone, I was secretly hoping that she would be the one. I knew that she liked the Creston area, and I was sure she would give serious consideration to coming back after graduation. She had literally beamed when I made that proposal to her on her final day here. All this week I'd been thinking of calling her—I would do it tonight.

Margaret Berg looked nervous as Doris went over the front-desk procedures with her. She had already spent an hour learning how to fold drapes and run the autoclave. Just when she was trying to process where to put all of the surgical packs and instruments, Doris moved on to the next task.

I was antsy this morning. Having someone new learning the ropes always made me uneasy. Doris and Shirley had been around me long enough to know how I liked things done, and being a creature of habit, I wanted things in the office to be the same from one day to the next.

I was avoiding the real reason I was so anxious. I had finally gotten up the courage to phone Marcie, and after a pleasant enough conversation, she told me that she'd decided not to come back to work for me. I wondered if she could tell by the sound of my voice just how disappointed I was.

First thing this morning, I had phoned the administration office at the vet college in Saskatoon and booked a time to hold interviews with students. I was told that it would be announced in one of the classes later in the morning. If I hadn't made the arrangements right then, I know I would have chickened out and plunged on alone.

I listened in as Margaret fielded her first call as receptionist. "Hello…Yes, sorry, it is the veterinary clinic…Oh, it's you, Morris. How are you doing? And how is Dianne?…The kids? Donnie's sleeping better at night now?…Oh yes, I just started today and I'm afraid I'm not up to speed on things yet."

She stood there with a look of concentration, then grabbed the daybook and started turning pages. "Uh huh, uh huh…No, he couldn't do it on Wednesday, but we can put you down for Thursday. Right…you take care now, Morris…but it sounds like you should be in bed with a cold like that. Okay…okay…good-bye." She hung up and made a notation in the book.

The day moved thankfully along at a leisurely pace, and it seemed as though Margaret was getting into the swing of things. Doris was on the phone; my neophyte assistant was helping to vaccinate a raucous Dalmatian puppy. Margaret's love for the pet had come through with the first, "Oh, isn't he the most gorgeous thing!" and continued while I trimmed his needle-sharp claws and listened to his chest. She was a natural with animals and put this puppy instantly at ease.

At that moment, the door burst open. I heard the most plaintive meow and a woman's trembling voice. "Easy, Gypsy…there's a girl. We're here now, Gypsy. Hold on now."

"I can manage here, Margaret—go see what's happening."

I injected the vaccine in the puppy's flank and administered a dose of worming medication before hurrying to see what was going on up front.

Margaret was standing with a middle-aged woman. Their attention was on a cardboard box that was slathered in blood.

"Oh, the poor thing…I'd just put her out of her misery," Margaret counselled.

"You would?" The woman's eyes filled with tears.

"I had an old tomcat something like this last summer. He got run over by a car outside my house and was dragging himself off the road. I ran to the garage for a hammer and just put him away."

I cringed at the graphic description. "Margaret!"

"Oh, look," she rattled on, "her guts are hanging out."

"Margaret." The tone of my voice got her attention. I shook my head resolutely. She opened her mouth as if to speak and then looked away.

"Have you any idea what happened?" I asked the woman.

"My son's visiting me from Lethbridge," she sobbed. "He had just pulled into the yard, and the moment he opened the car door his dog attacked Gypsy…I didn't even get to say hello—"

The cat let out a mournful yowl and stood erect, leaving a trail of fresh blood on the side of the box. She gave her owner a pleading look and flopped onto her side.

"Oh, Gypsy…" The woman dissolved in tears.

I picked up the box and maneuvered around the counter where Doris was finishing off the vaccination certificate.

"Look at—" Margaret began.

"Hold the box, Margaret, please," I said.

She held onto the sides of the carton as I lifted the cat onto the table. My newest assistant glanced furtively in my direction, now afraid to open her mouth. The cat meowed plaintively, slowly kneading her hind legs as if seeking a more comfortable position.

"There's a girl, Gypsy…Just keep her from backing up," I directed Margaret.

I quickly appraised the situation. The cat's gums were still faintly pink, and although her heart was racing, her femoral pulse was strong. I prodded along the animal's spine searching for the track mark that had been left by the dog's canine teeth. I gently probed the right side where the skin was perforated. Margaret was right—bowel was protruding, and more intestine bulged underneath the skin. I checked the scraped skin on the opposite side where the dog's teeth had skidded along when the jaw clamped shut.

Doris handed me the patient record. I glanced at the name—Gladys Truman.

"I guess we need some direction, Mrs. Truman. Gypsy has certainly been traumatized. I can't give you any guarantees, but I think we can save her."

"Oh, Doctor," Mrs. Truman gushed, "do what you can. My husband died in July of a heart attack…Gypsy was his cat. Since Jim's been gone, that cat hardly leaves my side. Bill was in tears when I left—totally beside himself that his own dog would attack his father's cat."

"We'll need an IV, Doris…Hold her here, Margaret."

Doris returned in a jiffy with all the fixings. Within five minutes, an intravenous was running and Gypsy was pre-medicated for surgery. I wasn't sure as the cat became sedated whether Margaret realized that it was the drug at work. I thought I could almost detect an "I told you so" look.

She watched as Doris and I anesthetized and prepared our patient for the procedure. She hardly spoke a word while I cleaned the wound and amputated a two-inch section of intestine. I had the bowel reconnected and replaced in the abdomen and the muscles of the flank repaired before she spoke.

"Do you really think she'll live?"

"I'll put money on it," I replied with a smile. I was happy with the way things had gone.

"I can't imagine doing all that for a cat," Margaret muttered.

"I would have done it for a hamster or a rat if it really was important to someone."

My *de facto* farmer gave me a look of horror.

"One thing you have to understand when you're working for me, Margaret. I spent seven years in university to learn to save animals in distress. I didn't go to learn how to swing a hammer."

The woman squirmed. "Don't get me wrong, Dave. I like animals and want to help them. I just don't like to see them suffer."

"I know, Margaret. You're a typical farmer…but you do me a favour. I want you to look after this cat until she's recovered. I want you to hold her and feed her her first meal, and I want you to be the one to discharge her to Mrs. Truman."

"But—" Margaret stammered.

"You got that, Doris?" Doris smiled and nodded.

"After you do that and watch Mrs. Truman with her cat, then you tell me whether this was worthwhile or not."

Doris and I hung close when Gypsy started growling and kneading her front paws. When she sat up on her sternum, I winked at Doris and we left her in Margaret's care.

It was three days later that she discharged Gypsy. Mrs. Truman and her son waited expectantly as Margaret carried the cat to the waiting room.

"Oh, Gypsy! I've missed you so much. You are such a pretty girl," Mrs. Truman crooned. She tenderly reached out for the cat and cradled her in her arms. Bill knelt beside his mother and stroked the animal's head and ran his fingers over her denuded flank. He straightened and took a half step in Margaret's direction.

"Thank you so much!" he exclaimed. "I can't tell you how grateful I am to all of you."

Margaret flushed. After the Trumans had gone, she said, "They were sure happy to get their cat back." She hesitated a moment as if calculating what she was about to say.

"I'm glad you were able to save her," she allowed. "You know, when I was a kid on the farm, I spent the whole time outside helping Dad. We had lots of animals around, and it seemed that there was always one getting sick. Dad was from Missouri and didn't have much to do with farming before he bought that section of land in Saskatchewan. There were no vets back then. I just accepted it as a fact of life that when something bad happened to the animals, we did away with them."

I nodded. "I appreciate that."

"Boy, did you see Mrs. Truman's eyes when she saw that cat? I can't believe how they lit up."

"They sure did, didn't they?"

Margaret was pretty well broken in by the time I headed to Saskatchewan. I was uneasy as I pulled away from the clinic and pointed my vehicle east toward Cranbrook. This was only the second time that I had left my practice in the care of another veterinarian. Sid was in his late fifties and had recently sold his own practice. I had hired him once before when I attended a veterinary convention.

It was unsettling to watch one of my clients follow another veterinarian into the exam room—sort of like sending your girlfriend off to the arms of another man.

The back of my Volkswagen was loaded down with boxes of apples and winter pears for Marcie, Cory, and a few of the professors I wanted to visit. I had intended to get away earlier, but just had to stay on to give last-minute instructions to clients. Now that I was free, it felt good to hit the road. I fantasized that as soon as I had another veterinarian working with me, I'd be able to do this often.

I found driving long distances therapeutic—maybe because it required some focus on immediate details, but left enough leeway for my mind to be somewhere else. It had seemed of late that "somewhere else" was a good place for my mind to be. As the Rockies came into view, I was drawn back to the Hurfords' cows.

I hated my complicity in the problems at Tsolum Farms. I just couldn't wrap my mind around the fact that my recommendations had brought such pain to a family that I had grown close to. In the final shakedown, six cows had died and fifty-six had been sent to slaughter because their udders were permanently damaged.

Although I berated myself for being so slow to twig to the diagnosis, I took some solace from the fact that the product had been distributed across North America and had been causing the same problems wherever it was in use. The fact that no other veterinarian had made the link to the source of the outbreak made me feel somewhat less like a failure.

But my role in this fiasco continued to nag at me—especially when the company had done nothing to stand behind its product. How an international drug company of its stature could fall back on archaic regulations to cover its ass was beyond me. Their field representatives continued to reassure me that the company would do the right thing, but the head office executives barraged me with babble about how laws in the United States and Canada only required sterility for a parenteral product. By definition, that was a product that was introduced directly into the body. They argued on a technicality that a product introduced into the mammary gland was not parenteral—like the uterus, the udder had a big cavern that was not really part of the body itself.

I was seething after my conversations with the company and nagged the Hurfords not to allow themselves to be taken advantage of. A few days ago, two Canadian representatives of the corporation appeared on their doorstep at ten o'clock at night. After ranting about the battery of high-powered lawyers on staff, they made Herb an offer of $21,000 and told him to settle—or he would be a very bitter man by the time the dust had settled.

Fortunately, Herb let little dust settle on these short-sighted executives before he threw them out into the night. He phoned me in a quandary the moment they left. How could they have done such a stupid thing? How could I have been a representative of a company that cared so little about doing the *right* thing?

I got a call the following morning that they wanted a meeting with me before leaving town. I joined them for breakfast at the Hacienda Inn, where they had spent the night. It wasn't hard to spot them—they were the only ones in the restaurant with double-breasted suits. To be honest, they were the only suits in town.

The waitress asked if I wanted my usual. I nodded, studying the two men. The older man forced a smile, then introduced himself and his younger, more dapper companion.

"Your client proved to be a bit difficult—" he began.

"I would hope so," I replied.

"What do you mean by that?" The young man raised his eyebrows—taken aback.

I didn't like this man. Just the look of him had my heart pounding. I knew my face was taking on the usual crimson glow.

"Well, if I were Herb, and you showed up at my place in the middle of the night and offered me $21,000 for sixty-two milking cows, you wouldn't be sitting at this table right now."

"That's pretty loose talk. I would think you'd advise your client to be sensible—to take a reasonable offer and get on with his life."

"You have no idea what this man's been through, have you?" I hesitated and struggled for words. "You don't give a tinker's damn what we've all been through. You show up in your pinstripe suit and look down your nose at us. People like you turn my stomach!"

I jumped to my feet. Silverware and dishes rattled. Coffee spilled. Both men stared at me in disbelief. I glared back.

"I can bet you've never spent any time on the road with your company."

The dapper fellow replied tersely, "I have an M.B.A. I started in management."

"That's obvious. Next time, pay attention to your field reps. If you'd bothered to consult with them, you wouldn't have pulled the stunt you did. There isn't a one of them that would have made as big an ass of himself as you two did."

Both men flushed. I turned to leave, then hesitated. "I'll do everything in my power to make you pay my client for what he lost…and I'll replace every one of your products on my shelf with those of a company that'll stand behind what it produces."

The waitress arrived with our orders.

"I suppose you expect us to pay for your breakfast!" spurted the dapper man.

"I expect nothing from you." I waited at the counter until my waitress arrived and paid my own account.

I rehashed the unsettling meeting as I drove through the windy Crowsnest Pass, imagining the many things I'd like to have said.

The scenery in the pass was magnificent. I tried to think of something pleasant. I chuckled at the memory of John Partington answering his door at two in the morning on Halloween night. David Hurford and I had ended our trick-or-treat rounds on his doorstep. I'm not sure why he acted so disgruntled when he dropped a withered apple into each of our bags—he was a dairy-man and would be getting up for milking in a couple of hours any-way. I admit it was rather unusual for me to be on his farm clad in a diaper. Some people just don't have a sense of humour.

It was on the freeway to Calgary that I saw the first signs to Taber. I had been hoping for a short visit with Brian, but it was already getting late—Cory was expecting me and I hated to keep him up past midnight. Until the last moment, I considered the stop. The final exit sign flashed like a neon sign as I continued on.

Poor Brian…I had gotten a letter from him last month and he sounded so unhappy. He was certain that his foster parents had taken him on simply to do farm labour. He bemoaned the fact that they refused to let him take a bus to Calgary to visit with John and wouldn't let him stay after school for sports.

I called him on receipt of the letter. In hushed tones, he spoke about how much he hated babysitting the couple's two children—and how much he missed everything in Creston.

"Can you go see Kenny?" he asked. "Can you see if Martha will take me back?"

Brian had thought the world of his caseworker from social services. Ken Blair had been raised in Casino just up the road from me. He was the sort of guy who really cared for his charges and had been supportive of the boys every step of the way. I had indeed discussed the situation with Ken and Martha. Martha, of course, said she would be more than happy to have the boy back. Ken had already placed a call to his counterpart in Taber, and the wheels were slowly grinding toward Brian's return. It'd be good to have the boy back. I missed him.

Although the roads were bare and dry all the way to Saskatoon, it was close to twelve local time when I pulled into the apartment complex where Cory lived.

"Well, it's damn time you got here," he said, greeting me at the door. "What took you so long?"

"You know me—had trouble getting out of there."

"Sit down…Want a beer?"

"Sure thing."

By the end of the third beer, I had caught up on all the gossip at the vet college. Cory had a new perspective now that he was a resident, and it was interesting to hear how the political landscape had changed since my departure from the ivory tower.

"So, what are you looking for in a student?" he asked.

"Well, if I had my druthers, she'd be five ten, in her mid-twenties, and be an experienced raft racer."

"Have you asked her yet?"

"Yeah."

"Nothing doing?"

"Apparently not. It sounded good when she left in August, but she seemed to cool off. I called her a couple of weeks ago, and she said she'd decided against it…Called her again last night to see if she wanted some apples. Sort of hoped she would have changed her mind, but no dice."

"Too bad. You two seemed to have something cooking."

"I thought so, too." I downed the rest of my beer and grabbed another. "But you know that I was never much on dealing with women. I seem to do really well with mother figures. Our old landlady used to just love me, and I've got several more in Creston who think I'm the cat's meow."

I spent the morning distributing apples and visiting with old acquaintances. After a few hours the fuzziness from the beer the night before wore off. I showed up in the seminar room that had been assigned to me for interviews. I was surprised at the interest and had highlighted several candidates I thought would fit in well with the plans I had for the future of Creston Veterinary Clinic.

There were eight candidates, and the interviews took most of the afternoon. One applicant from Lethbridge had a particular interest in horses. He was personable and I thought he would fit in well with the staff and my clients. I was already thinking he would be the one, and I asked if I could contact him later in the evening.

I was heading out the door with my notebook in hand when Cory walked in.

"Well, you ready to head for supper?" I asked.

"No, I'm here for my interview."

"You? Are you serious?"

He nodded.

"Why didn't you mention you were interested earlier? It would have saved me a trip out here."

"I guess I just made up my mind."

"Well…when can you start?"

The Hunter's Dilemma

"She's in terrible shape, Dave." The tall, lean man rushed past me as I opened the door.

"Where do you want her?" he asked, delicately cradling his burden. His face was flushed and deep lines creased his forehead as he peered down at his pet.

"Right in there." I motioned him toward the stainless-steel table in the back room.

"I swear this morning she was as good as gold, and now look at her…She can hardly hold her head up."

Marty pushed his cowboy hat to the back of his head and gently unwrapped the woollen blanket from around his dog. The Boston terrier was indeed in terrible straits. Barely able to keep herself upright, her breaths came in short, choppy bursts.

"Do you think she's having a heart attack?" Marty's hand trembled as his callused fingers stroked the sleek head of his beloved pet. "I feel so helpless."

I knelt next to the table for a closer look at Sophie. She certainly wasn't herself. A delightfully social animal, she would ordinarily be crawling all over me in an attempt to wash me with her long pink tongue.

"Come here, Sophie." My encouragement induced only the slightest twitch of the crinkled vestige that was her tail.

"I've never seen her like this." Marty shrugged his shoulders. "You know her…she hardly ever holds still."

I gently slid the dog closer to the edge of the table. Her body felt ice cold.

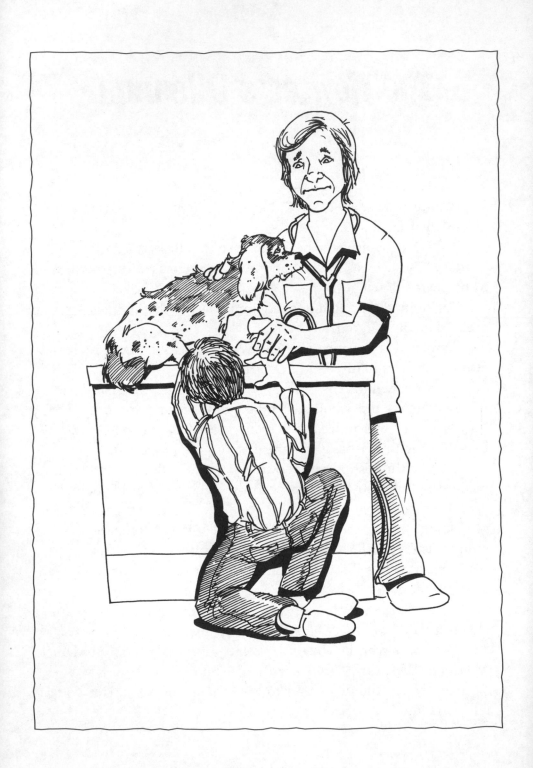

"Oh, Sophie, you poor thing." Grabbing a thermometer, I shook it down and inserted it into her rectum. I rolled back her jowl to get a look at her mucous membranes. The normally pink lips and gums were pale. Small bruises marred the gum line, and on her right lip I noticed one the size of a quarter.

"Is there any chance she could have gotten into mouse poison, Marty?"

The man blanched as he focused his blue eyes intently on my face. "God, yes. I put some out at the shop just last week. One of those damned pack rats moved in—can't stand the smell of those critters—so I put some way back under the workbench. I didn't think she'd go there, but it sure is possible." He looked woefully in my direction. "Do you think she could have gotten into that stuff?"

I lifted Sophie's eyelids one at a time. Her mucous membranes were white. Tiny bruises, popcorn-kernel size, dotted the whites of her eyes.

"I think there's a very good chance she did," I responded.

I removed the thermometer. The base was covered with dark pasty blood. Her temperature was 36.4, more than two degrees below normal. I lifted her leg and ran my hand over the smooth inner thigh—bruises everywhere.

"Oh, Sophie, what have I done to you?" Marty moaned.

I quickly put together the materials I'd need to start an intravenous drip. Marty seemed distressed when I drove the sharp tip of the administration set into the one-litre bag of fluids. He looked away as saline filled the line and slowly displaced the air. I ripped off a couple of pieces of adhesive tape, stuck them on the edge of the table, then grabbed a gauze and soaked it with alcohol. Applying a tourniquet to Sophie's elbow, I rubbed her foreleg aggressively in an attempt to build a vein. Her master stared at the ceiling as I tore back the cellophane packaging of the catheter.

"Just hold her head," I instructed.

I drove the needle into the ripple that was the vein. Watery-looking blood oozed into the catheter. I flexed the dog's leg, working it back and forth to get enough blood to fill a tiny pair of blue-topped capillary tubes. I noted the time, connected the intra-venous, and taped the apparatus to her leg.

Marty's complexion was wan. Staring at the exit, he had the most distant, forlorn look on his face.

I grabbed my stethoscope and listened intently to the sound of Sophie's chest. Her heart rate was rapid; the lung sounds seemed increased. I was praying that her airways were not totally flooded with blood.

"I don't need to tell you how serious this is, Marty. There's an antidote to warfarin, but all it does is compete with the poison—it takes time to work."

I calculated her weight and the dose of vitamin K that we would need. Marty looked away again as I drew the medication into a syringe and injected it at several different sites under the dog's skin.

"There's a girl. Good girl, Sophie." The dog didn't flinch.

I rotated the blue-top tubes back and forth to check them and noted that the blood still flowed as freely as when I put it in.

"What are you looking for?" Marty asked.

"Ordinary blood would have clotted by now. It's rare to have it take more than six minutes after collection."

"What was that stuff you gave her?"

"Vitamin K—it allows her to start make clotting factors again…The problem is, she needs them now. You can see that she's bleeding everywhere. The only way we'll be able to stop it is to give her blood that has clotting factors in it."

"You mean transfuse her?"

I nodded. "I'd be afraid to try and get her through it without a transfusion. If I were a betting man, I'd wager on the side of the poison."

"Well, let's do whatever we have to. I don't want to lose her if there's something we can possibly do."

"I usually use my own dog as a donor, but we collected from Lug just last week. Do you know of another critter we could use?"

Marty thought for a moment. "My brother has a couple of big dogs. I'm sure Oscar would let me bring in Trooper."

"Well, why don't you get on the phone and make the arrangements. We don't have much time."

I wrapped Sophie in her blanket and got her settled in a kennel in the surgery. I had just finished filling a couple of gallon jugs with hot water when Marty rushed back in.

"I'll go and get Trooper now. Oscar says it's all right with him."

I puttered around the office getting things ready as I waited for his return. I had the collection apparatus all laid out. I considered giving Doris a call—it sure didn't hurt to have an extra set of hands around when collecting blood. I picked up the phone. Oh heck, Marty and I could manage—Doris had little enough opportunity to get away from this place.

I checked Sophie again. Her breathing seemed more laboured. It may have been the stress of the hospitalization or being locked up all alone, but I didn't like the looks of her. I listened again—her lung sounds were definitely worse. I stretched a sheet of plastic over the inside of the kennel door to create a tent and inserted the hose from the anesthetic machine between the bars. I turned on the oxygen and cranked up the flow.

I was thankful to see Marty back inside half an hour with the borrowed dog. The way Sophie was looking, I was beginning to panic. The blood in the capillary tubes had still not clotted, and I had no doubt that we were treating a dog in the advanced stage of warfarin toxicity.

"Right on the table there, Marty. We better get this show on the road."

Trooper was a heavy-set springer spaniel. Oversized for his breed and in top condition, he appeared to be an ideal candidate for a blood donor. According to my records, we had seen him twice—both times for his annual vaccinations.

The robust dog whined and nervously surveyed the room as he was deposited on the stainless-steel surface. Shivering convulsively, he glared at Marty, then shot a worried look in my direction.

"I'm afraid I'll have to shave him a bit to find a vein."

Marty nodded and studied the corner of the room as I fired up the clippers and removed a narrow strip of hair directly over the cephalic vein.

"Just hold his head up against your chest."

I threaded Trooper's foot through a tourniquet, tightened it over his elbow, and wiped down the foreleg with alcohol.

"There's a boy, Trooper."

I pulled the plastic guard from the needle of the collection apparatus with my teeth. Lining up the large-bore needle, I drove it into the centre of the vein. Blood flowed down the transparent plastic tube and disappeared out of sight over the rim of the table. The dog's eyes bugged as he attempted to see what I had just done to him.

"It's okay, Trooper, you're doing just fine."

I held his foreleg firmly at the elbow while flexing and massaging his foot. Blood flowed freely from the end of the tube to mingle with the anticoagulant in the transfusion bag. I stepped on the container repeatedly to facilitate the mixing and continued to work the animal's foot back and forth to maintain a steady flow.

"You really are a trooper, aren't you, fellow? Nothing to this...Are you okay, Marty?"

The man was sweating profusely, and his cowboy hat was perched precariously on the back of his head. His eyes were closed; his body swayed ever so slightly. The knuckles of the fingers that held Trooper's head were devoid of colour.

"I don't feel so good," he replied blandly.

"I can see that. Take a deep breath. You'll be all right."

I knew I was lying the moment the words left my mouth. I reached up and grabbed Trooper just in time. Marty's hat toppled to the floor as he leaned against the wall. He opened his eyes for a moment and stared blankly at the ceiling, then crumpled into a heap on the floor.

"Easy, Trooper. Good boy."

I struggled to hold the dog's leg in a prone position and keep the collection going. Stepping over Marty's body, I attempted to draw Trooper against me. He jerked his leg and the needle pulled out. I grabbed the apparatus before it hit the floor and worked to keep the dog on the table. What I wouldn't do for another hand. Blood oozed from the puncture site on Trooper's forearm. When I reached to put pressure on it, he panicked and jumped to the floor.

"Don't feel too good," Marty mumbled.

"Thank God, you're still in the land of the living."

He lifted his head, rested it against the wall, and moaned. "I must have passed out...never happened before. I go hunting all the time...can gut an animal and never feel the least bit queasy. I don't believe this."

I left the hunter muttering about his expeditions and chased Trooper to the exit. The poor dog's eyes brimmed with anticipation as I scooped him up. Putting pressure on his foreleg, I returned him to the table.

"Oh man, look at his leg!" Marty averted his eyes from the sight of the blood.

I smiled ruefully. "Do you think you can hold him while I clean him up? The needle pulled out when you fainted...Just look away while I do the washing."

"Not a problem," the man affirmed. "Don't know what went wrong with me." He managed to get back on his feet and lean unsteadily against the table. "I'll be fine...really."

I returned with a bowl of cold water from the surgery and scrubbed at the blood that had soaked into the thick hair and the feathering at the back of the dog's leg. Marty held Trooper loosely to his chest. As I washed down the blood, I did my best to keep the bowl from the man's direct line of vision.

"Do you think you're up for another go, or should I call some-one else in for help?"

"Hell no, don't bother anyone else! I'm fine. That's never hap-pened to me before…I'll be just fine."

I clipped a strip of hair from Trooper's right leg, taking great pains to make it even with the other side. "Got to make sure your racing stripes match, old boy."

Marty had a look of conviction on his face as I picked up the apparatus and again drove the needle into the vein. He stared directly at it—determined to prove that it didn't bother him.

"Good boy, Trooper."

It wasn't long before my helper's eyes began to take on that far-off look. I got hold of Trooper's head just as Marty let it go. His knees buckled and he sank once more to the floor. Clutching the edge of the table, he struggled to his knees.

"I can do this," he insisted.

I could hardly hear him. I was clinging desperately to Trooper's leg. The dog pulled back, teetering dangerously close to the edge of the table.

"Easy, boy. You stay put a few more minutes and this'll all be over."

Like a punch-drunk fighter unwilling to admit defeat, Marty dragged himself erect, reached out, and pulled the dog to him. As the two swayed back and forth, it was hard to determine who was holding up whom. The blood was still flowing, and the bag was beginning to appear slightly rounded. It wasn't half full yet, but it may well have been enough to mean the difference between life and death for my patient.

"Are you okay, Marty?"

He didn't answer—just stood stock-still, as if in a catatonic state. His eyes were closed; his face was ashen. I maneuvered around the table, taking care to maintain my grip on the dog's leg. With the tip of my toe, I dragged the bag to where I could see it. I stroked Trooper's head and tried to extricate him from my assis-tant's fingers.

"Marty...Marty! Maybe you better sit down."

Without a hint of a verbal response, he sank to the floor. I drew Trooper against my stomach. Holding him with my right hand, I squeezed his toes with my left. The needle and tubing perched precariously in place.

"There's a boy, just a little more blood for Sophie."

I had no idea whether or not the blood was still running. For all I knew now, the line had clotted and I was just wasting my time. Oh, that this could be as easy as a human collection—in the cloistered environment of human medicine, all the nurse had to do was hit a big vein and tell her patient to lie still. If the flow decreased or wasn't great to start with, she might ask him to clench and relax his hand. There was no juggling, no wrestling, no fainting helper. Hell, they could handle half a dozen patients at once. I seemed incapable of managing one.

"I can gut a deer." The statement was barely audible. My assistant's face was still flat to the floor.

"Are you with us again, Marty?"

"Hunt all the time...I can gut a deer."

"I know, Marty, I know."

By the time he had risen to his hands and knees, I was convinced that the line had clotted. The collection bag had looked the same size for the last five minutes, and I was darned if I could see any signs of the blood flowing into the neck.

"How you feeling there, champ?"

"I'm fine now." From a kneeling position, he grabbed onto the table and slowly pulled his lanky frame erect.

"Do you think you can hold onto Trooper for me?"

"Sure thing."

Trooper's tail wiggled in anticipation at his "uncle's" approach. The dog had had about enough of this foolishness; the expression on his face left little doubt that he was expecting to be rescued. I relinquished my hold on him and picked up the blood bag. Just as I suspected, the flow had stopped.

"Damn!"

"Troubles?" Marty's voice was distant.

"Yes, our line has clotted. A dog has a much smaller vein to collect from when compared to a human. That's why I have to keep massaging the lower limb to keep the blood flowing. Otherwise, it slows down and clots before it gets to the anticoagulant in the bag."

"I guess I'm not a very good assistant," he mused. "Can't understand it."

"Well, we'll have one last go at it."

I placed a gauze over the puncture site and withdrew the needle. As Marty held the dog, I began working on the collection apparatus to free the line of clots. Spurt after spurt of gelatinous debris shot from the needle and plopped onto the table.

Marty stood like a statue. His eyes were closed as he mechanically massaged Trooper's floppy ears. I chased the last of the clots from the end of the needle and filled the line with anticoagulant-laden blood.

"We're ready, Marty."

He opened his eyes momentarily and gave me a meek smile. "I can do this," he whispered to himself.

"We have to use a back leg now." I clipped a small square over the hock and extended the dog's leg. Rubbing with an alcohol swab, I raised the vein and glanced at my helper. His face was still waxen, and I had no reason to hope that he would be any more stable this time than the last.

"Let's do this for Sophie, Marty. This vein is going to be harder to work with than the front one. You try your best to stay with me."

I slipped the needle into the vein where it crossed over the hock. Fresh blood began to flow, and I watched as it pushed a bubble of air down the tubing and into the bag. Slowly massaging Trooper's foot, I kept my eye on the receptacle.

Regardless of how much we got this time, I'd start the transfusion as soon as the flow stopped. What we had collected already was probably enough to get Sophie back on track, and each moment we fooled with this procedure was a moment the dog could ill afford.

Marty's face was pallid. His eyes were clamped shut; his hands were draped loosely over Trooper's shoulders. If he could only stay with me for a bit longer…

"There's a boy, Trooper," I chimed. "You're being such a good fellow."

I squeezed the dog's toes and viewed with satisfaction the steady flow of blood into the bag. Marty began a rhythmic swaying action as he battled to stay erect.

"I can gut a deer," he mumbled.

"You sure can, Marty…and you can do this."

The man's face contorted and he sank to his knees.

"Easy, Trooper…there's a good dog." I stopped massaging and held him down on the table. Marty's hands remained on the spaniel's shoulder. His forehead rested half on the table edge, half on Trooper's neck. "You still with me, Marty?"

There was a wiggling of a finger, a whitening of knuckles as he maintained his precarious position.

"Way to go…just hold him still."

I returned to my post and resumed the firm squeezing and milking of Trooper's foot. Gazing in wonderment at Marty, I was amazed that he was still hanging in. He mumbled something totally unintelligible.

"Couldn't make that out, Marty. You doing okay?"

"I can gut a deer," he muttered.

"Yes, and you can do a damned fine job of holding a dog for a transfusion."

By the time the flow of blood stopped, the bag was distended and I was getting more and more anxious to get on with the transfusion. After all, the objective of this exercise was not to fill this bag, but to save Marty's beloved Sophie.

I removed the collection needle and taped a gauze in place. "We're done!"

There was not the slightest reaction from the man as I pried his fingers from Trooper's hair coat and carried him to a kennel in the back room. When I left him, Marty was balancing precariously on his knees with his forehead still resting on the edge of the tabletop.

Connecting the administration set, I rushed into the surgery and set up the transfusion. It was with a sense of accomplishment that I watched the drip, drip, drip of the blood in the filtration chamber.

Sophie coughed, and blood-tinged fluid appeared on the edge of her nostrils. I prayed that we had gotten to her in time.

When I returned to the examination room, Marty lay stretched out on the floor, his hands under his head like a sleeping child. He actually looked relaxed.

"Are you all right, Marty?"

He stirred and propped himself up on his elbow. "Oh man, I feel like I've been run over by a truck." He pulled himself to a seated position, resting his head against the wall. "You know, I've been hunting for years and seen all sorts of blood and guts. I never thought something like this could bother me until today."

"It might just have to do with seeing blood from animals you care about."

He smiled sheepishly, dragging himself to an erect position. "God, if Oscar finds out, I'll never hear the end of it."

I smiled back. "I guess there's no reason for him to ever find out."

Within several hours, it was obvious that Sophie had passed the crisis. Her breathing gradually became relaxed, and I removed the supplemental oxygen. When I went to bed that night, she was a tired little dog with bruises from one end of her body to the other. It had been nip and tuck, and although she might not feel it at the moment, she was one lucky pooch.

By the time we discharged Sophie the next afternoon, she had regained most of her vim and vigour. As I handed her to Marty, she squirmed and struggled to wash his face with her tongue.

"Sorry I was such a pain," he apologized, trying without much conviction to control the wriggling dog.

"Well, it was one heck of an ordeal," I replied, "but looking at her now, it all seems worthwhile."

Marty smiled and headed for the door.

"Have a good weekend!" I hollered after him.

"I will! Oscar and I are going hunting in the morning."

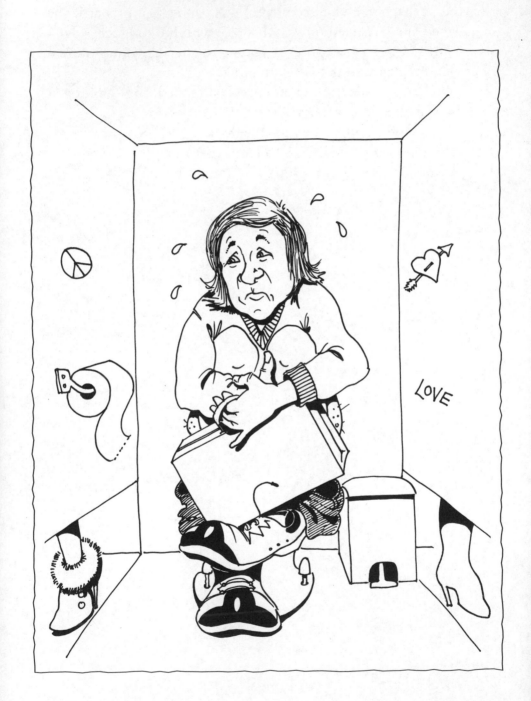

A Brief History of Timing

"Dr. Perrin, this is Janet Schofer. Cliff and I need your help with a heifer." The woman was out of breath. I could just picture the slender blonde clad in gumboots and a bulky winter coat standing in the kitchen of her ranch-style home.

"Uh-h-h...Is she a good-size animal, Janet? Or will this be a Caesarian?" It was only a few minutes after six, and the woman's call had roused me from a sound sleep.

"It doesn't look good to me...She's pretty small. We had to chase her into the corral from the far end of the pasture. We tried to check her out there, but she just wouldn't hold still long enough for Cliff to find out what was going on. The calf's head has started through...The tongue is pretty swollen. Cliff tried to get hold of the feet, but he was only in there a few minutes before he said to call you."

"I'll get dressed and head out there."

"Cliff told me to ask you to hurry if you could. He thinks the calf's pretty weak."

I yanked on my long johns and heavy wool socks, then worked the legs of my blue jeans over them. Lug circled around me, constantly thrusting his nose into my hands to tell me he was ready for adventure.

"You sure you want to come? You could be sitting out in the car steaming up my windows for hours."

The big shepherd let out a howl and twirled around, whapping my legs with his tail.

"Okay, okay, you can come." I dug out a heavy sweatshirt and checked to make sure it was one with the sleeves cut off. I would need bare arms for the calving, and would usually be shirtless for the procedure. But in cold like this, I'd definitely want something warm against my upper body.

"Okay, mutt, let's go." Lug jumped up, licked my fingers, and tore off down the stairs. I detoured into the pharmacy for a new bottle of lidocaine. I had a feeling this excursion would involve surgery.

I shivered as I stepped out into the cool air. It was a blustery morning in early March, and winter seemed reluctant to relinquish its grip on the valley. The streetlights still glowed, but the dark of the night was already retreating. Fine particles of snow drifted to the sidewalk. A car roared past dragging a cloud of tiny flakes in its wake.

Lug headed for the parking lot at a run, stopping to lift a leg on all his favourite marking posts. I unlocked the vehicle, started the engine, and brushed the fine layer of snow from the hood and windows of the car.

"Come on, boy, hurry up." The dog tore toward me, then hesitated, lifted his tail, and squatted for a quick dump. I've always admired a dog's sense of timing. A vision of Janet and Cliff waiting anxiously next to their labouring heifer flashed through my mind. As if sensing my anxiety, Lug finished his duties and dove in through the open car door, taking up his position as co-pilot.

The Schofer farm was only a few miles from Creston, just off Highway 3 on the flat land. The car heater was barely discharging a hint of warm air by the time we pulled into the drive. I drove past the feedlot and parked at a gate next to their machine shop. Lug peered through the side window and whined excitedly as Janet puffed her way from the house with a pail of steaming water suspended from each hand.

"Hello, Dr. Perrin. Thanks for getting here so quickly."

"No problem."

I gathered together the materials I would need for a calving on the chance that the offspring could be delivered naturally. I passed the buckets of water over the gate to Janet and climbed over myself, balancing my calving jack and bucket on the top rail. Following her down the alleyway between the feedlot and the paddock that housed the pregnant cows, I took a last look back at Lug, whose nose was pressed to the windshield. How he'd love to be in on the action.

Janet's pace was brisk and we had soon covered the hundred-yard distance to the enclosure where the heifer was confined. Stopping at a rail fence, the slender woman hefted the buckets of water and passed them one at a time to her husband on the other side. Cliff's face was clouded with frustration, and he wasn't in the mood for pleasantries.

As I struggled up with my equipment, Janet climbed over the fence and disappeared into the calving shed. The number of times that the Schofers shinnied over these structures in a day, it was no wonder that neither carried an extra pound of fat between them.

"Doggone it, anyway. Things were going so well up till now," Cliff sighed. "Couldn't seem to get hold of those feet at all. I don't think there's much room in there." He grabbed the bucket that contained the chains and Bridine soap.

In the centre of a circle of light shining from an overhead bulb was a squat Hereford heifer. She stood in exhausted resignation, tied with a rope halter to a cross rail in the ten-by-ten pen. Her ears drooped; her back was hunched. She pushed weakly against a pink blob that protruded from her vagina. Moisture clung to the long, curly red hair that stood up on her back, and steam rose from her into the crisp morning air.

"Has she been steady on her feet?"

"Sure seemed steady when we chased her around the entire pasture. I tried checking her out there, but there was no way. Finally got Dad to come out with the pickup and herded her in here."

A short, balding man in his eighties perched on a hay bale in the corner of the enclosure. "You remember Dr. Perrin, Dad." The man pulled his wool toque further down his shiny head and nodded at me.

I scrubbed up the heifer's back end and the long pink membranes that hung from it, then slipped on a plastic sleeve and soaped it up. Turning my hand sideways, I slowly pressed forward into the vagina. I immediately ran into the calf's head and a swollen, protruded tongue.

"Do you think it's still alive, Dr. Perrin?"

I slipped my fingers into the calf's mouth and wiggled them around. The immediate, quick champ of its jaw gave me my answer.

"Yes, it's still alive," I said, pushing beyond the calf's head in search of its elusive feet. Janet and Cliff exchanged a glance, and Cliff broke into a tired smile. My hand came to an immediate halt as it jammed between the calf's neck and the heifer's pelvis. "There's no way we have enough room here for a natural delivery, though—barely enough for the head to come through on its own."

Cliff's smile faded. "I was afraid of that." He turned to his father. "Well, Dad, looks like you get to see your first Caesarian."

"If you want to get the extension cord ready for my clippers," I suggested, "I'll head back to get my instruments. We'll need a bale to put them on. And maybe you could shorten up the lead shank just a bit."

I hauled my calving jack and breech back to the car to replace them with surgical supplies. Lug anxiously awaited my return, his head bobbing back and forth over the dashboard, certain we were ready to move on.

"Settle down, you big boob. We're not done yet."

"Boy, you sure are shaving her bald." Cliff's father stood behind me as I stripped the last of the hair from the cow's flank and began focusing on the ridge over the base of her tail. "Why are you shaving her so far back? You don't have to cut her there, do you?"

"No. There won't be any cutting back here, but I do need to disinfect this whole area before I freeze her. We'll give her a shot to deaden her back end and keep her from pushing." The senior Schofer nodded his head in acceptance, watching silently as I began scrubbing the animal's smoothly clipped side.

Cliff took off into the pasture for a quick check on the other cattle while Janet remained at my elbow to assist. I directed a twenty-gauge needle between the vertebrae of the cow's tail and slowly injected lidocaine until the tail flopped with a dead weight from side to side.

"Is that like a spinal in people?" Mr. Schofer queried.

"Exactly like it. But I'm only using this to deaden her pelvis and keep her from pushing. I'm going to block the nerves as they come off the spine to numb her side."

"Why's that?" Mr. Schofer was obviously enjoying the show.

"Well, I could do the procedure with a spinal just like in people, but if I did that, she wouldn't be able to stand up and it would make surgery more difficult."

The old man's eyes widened in disbelief. "You mean you aren't going to lay her down for this?"

I shook my head and filled a thirty-millilitre syringe with local anesthetic. The heifer flinched as I directed the two-inch needle to the level of the lumbar vertebra and injected the anesthetic. She kicked her foot in my direction, but with my butt planted firmly against her neck and front leg, I was out of her range. Repeating the procedure at several other sites, I leaned against her and waited for the freezing to take effect.

Moments later, the cow stood stock-still. My observer nodded his appreciation. He chirped on about a tough calving he'd seen back in the '50s as I prepared both the critter and myself for surgery. By the time I had the instruments laid out and my gown and surgery gloves on, he had dragged over a straw bale and arranged it carefully for a ringside seat. I welcomed the audience—his enthusiasm made for good company.

I clamped on a drape and made my first incision. Mr. Schofer watched in fascination as I cut through the animal's side and air rushed in to fill the vacuum.

"If that isn't the darndest thing!" He grinned as my arm disappeared into the animal's abdomen. "Who would ever have thought she'd just stand there and let you cut her open?"

The heifer shifted uncomfortably as I grasped the calf's hind feet and hefted them up into the incision site.

And that's when it happened.

I paused, my arms still half inside the animal. In fact, I must have paled, too, because Mr. Schofer's rapt attention shifted from the cow's open belly to my face. He searched my expression, trying to discern the reason for the change in my demeanour.

"Everything okay, Doctor?"

"Oh yeah. So far so good." But that was a bald-faced lie.

It wasn't the surgery—that had progressed as well as anyone could hope. No, the problem here was entirely with me. Or rather with last night's homemade baked beans. Because right then and there, nature was calling me—big time. And, unfortunately, I was staring into the open side of a client's cow. Now was certainly not the time to take a break of any kind. *Excuse me, everybody. Just swat the flies away from the gaping hole in your heifer while I wander off and take a dump.* In fact, the john was a good five-minute hike back to the house. So, with no other choice, I would apparently have to grin and bear it.

I gritted my teeth, determined to carry on, and thankfully the inopportune urge subsided. I was safe…for the moment. I smiled to reassure Mr. Schofer senior that all was well with the world of the country vet, and continued slicing through the uterus down the length of the calf's hind legs, prompting the pale caps of the calf's feet to come into view.

"So that's what the calf bed looks like from this side," the old man commented when I severed the uterine wall. "I've seen a few of 'em from the other side when they got pushed out by accident."

He was using the farmer's vernacular for the uterus, which did on occasion turn inside out (the way a shirtsleeve would) when a critter pushed too hard.

I pulled the calf up and out. It was a small baby. The heifer let out a long sigh as if in relief. At that point, I was more than a little envious of that heifer, who must have been feeling so much lighter and more satisfied. Now deposited at Janet's feet, the calf shook its head and peered uncertainly around.

"Can you open the suture material for me?" I asked Janet. It was time to close the heifer up again. Janet took the lid off the jar and held it out to me. I reached for a length of the catgut and....Oh no, not again.

It was worse this time—like a lead weight dropping through the pit of my bowels. The wave very nearly knocked me over.

Oh, my kingdom for a porta-potty. Clearly I'd underestimated Mother Nature. She was never one to abide by any man's schedule, and I was obviously no exception. A moment ago, I was a climber on Everest, certain I could outrun her storm; now I was ready to bow...or at least squat...at her almighty feet. I inhaled deeply. This time, Janet noticed something was awry. How could she not notice as the sweat ran down my forehead? I stood there paralyzed while she held out the suture material.

"Doctor Perrin?"

I tried my best to cover. "Just...a little emotional. Get that way at a birth sometimes."

Janet nodded, but she was clearly not convinced. I breathed in and out in short quick puffs, feeling all eyes on me. Hyperventilating provided some reprieve from the discomfort, but I knew time was running out.

I quickly grabbed a length of suture from the alcohol bath Janet still offered. I fumbled to attach it to a curved needle and started suturing with a vengeance. My hands couldn't stitch fast enough as the next painful peristaltic wave washed over me. My God, I suddenly thought, I couldn't be the only medical professional to be assaulted by such unfortunate timing. What does a brain surgeon do when a patient's skull lies open on the operating table and he suddenly has to lighten his load? How many poor bastards had lost their lives just because Doctor Whatsit was abruptly overcome by an overpowering need to trip down to the two-holer? And what about a prime minister or president? I would bet one leader of the free world or another had been struck dumb by a hurry-up call just as he was about to address the nation or make some snap judgement that could affect all humanity.

I managed to tie off the final suture pattern on the uterus. The heifer stood quietly, jaw clenched. I began wiping her down hastily, whistling some tuneless song to distract me from the torture that ravaged my gut.

Cliff had returned from his rounds, and he and Janet were fussing over their new bull-calf and drying it with towels. My octogenarian observer was all grins as he watched his son and daughter-in-law care for the calf. Smiling broadly, he shook his head. "Never would have believed you could just pull the calf out of her side with her standing there like that."

I was partway up on the closure of the peritoneum and the internal abdominal muscles when I was overcome with the feeling I wasn't going to make it. This successful operation was going to end in great embarrassment for me, I was sure. I closed my eyes and tensed every muscle in my body in a frantic attempt to stave off the impending catastrophe. In that instant, I flashed back to another time…not entirely unlike this one.

I was in Vancouver, halfway between my room at the Place Vanier dorms and the UBC library. It was pouring with rain and I was drenched. Although by this point of my stay in the rain capital of planet Earth, I had bought an umbrella, I still wouldn't be caught dead using it. Back home I had not once seen a man carry an umbrella!

Sloshing through puddles, I remembered arguing with myself about which way to head for the relief I was in desperate need of finding. It would be beyond humiliation to fill my drawers no matter where I was, but at least if that happened, I could choose to be on my way home. Instead, I held my breath, tucked my briefcase under my arm, and made a dash toward the library. I had midterms the next week, and I absolutely had to get my psychology term paper out of the way. A block from my destination, I set my briefcase down, doubled over, and clutched at my belly. I was certain my fate was sealed. For a moment, I considered just letting go and accepting the shame—I might just be able to get home without seeing anyone who knew me. I took a step in the direction of the dorm, then whirled around and hurried on to the library.

By the time I reached the stately stone building, I was close to despair. I waddled up the stairs and streaked in the direction of the posted lavatory signs. I crashed through the john door and raced for the only open stall in a string of four. I whipped down my pants and my butt hit the toilet seat—ice-cold porcelain relief. I'd made it! I closed my eyes, relaxed, and gave thanks for my deliverance.

It was a good minute later that I took stock of my surroundings. I couldn't put my finger on it—maybe it was the neatly scribed graffiti—but something felt just a little foreign. I checked under the stall to my left. What kind of a guy wore white rain boots? I looked under the stall to my right—beige rubbers with black fur trim. I quickly lifted my feet. My God, I was in the women's washroom!

My heart pounded. I wondered how many of the other occupants had picked up on the chick with the size 14 EEE running shoes. *Oh Lord, how could you have allowed this to happen?* The toilet to the left of me flushed. I heard the latch open and the door bang shut. I peeked warily through the crack. The nineteen-year-old female was standing just outside my cubicle, looking straight at it. She had a puzzled look on her plump face. She stooped forward to peer under. I grabbed my briefcase. Oh man, she had to know! She pushed hesitantly on my door.

My hand shot forward to reinforce the barrier between us. It contacted the metal surface with far more force than I intended. The door rattled noisily. I heard a stifled gasp; the woman in the white boots rushed for the exit. My legs ached from holding them off the ground. The toilet to my right flushed. I had to get out of there! Quickly hiking my pants, I zipped up. The neighbouring door opened. I again lifted my feet and balanced the briefcase on my lap. I'd make a break for it the moment this girl was gone.

I reached down to pull up on my knees—my calves and hamstrings ached from the effort. Through the crack in the door I could see the shapely blonde gazing at her reflection in the mirror. She applied lipstick, smacking her lips together and running her tongue over them before she finally puckered.

Come on, chicky-poo, can it and get out of here. She fluffed her hair with the back of a comb, then plucked a brush from the overstuffed handbag that lay on the counter. Surely to God she wasn't going to primp all day. She seemed to have enough inventory in that purse to keep her doing maintenance for hours. I was totally exasperated by the time she finally stuffed her implements back in her handbag and headed out the door.

I counted to ten before springing the latch and making a run for it. I reached the exit in just four paces. Hitting it on a dead run, I struggled to remember the lay of the land. I was pretty sure that a sharp turn to the left would get me to the main floor study area. Just a few more moments of embarrassment, and I could get my reference material and hide in some remote cubicle.

The door swung open, and I broke from my confinement into the hall like a Brahman bull exploding from a rodeo chute. I burst into a throng of female students who stood in a semi-circle around the door. I recognized the plump girl in the white boots. "There he is!" she said, pointing an accusatory finger right at me. "I saw his shoes…He's…"

The shock on every female face as I made my charge was evident. I extended my briefcase as a battering ram and broke through their ranks. My left arm was raised instinctively to my face in an attempt to hide my features. How could they ever forget what this gangly giant looked like? How could I ever show my face again, knowing that I was some sort of pervert in the eyes of all the women on campus?

I veered right toward the exit and hit the crash bars with a force that sent an echo throughout the entire antechamber. I charged past a woman sheathing her umbrella and plummeted down the stairs, three at a time. I was a block away from the library before I slowed my pace and the panic began to subside. I tipped my head back, relishing the pounding of the rain on my face. My term paper would have to wait.

I wondered if Cliff's father could see how red my ears were— just thinking about that day six long years before had refreshed the blush. I tried to remind myself how insignificant the pains had seemed after my episode in the women's washroom—it was all a matter of perspective.

Pressing on with the suturing, I reached the top of the first layer and pushed against the heifer's side to expel as much air as possible. This was the point where I usually lifted my knee under the critter's tummy where I elevated and compressed the abdominal contents to get rid of as much dead space as possible. Right at the moment, there was no way on God's green earth that I'd do anything that involved parting my cheeks!

I raced down the outer layer of the muscle closure, whipping back and forth with continuous sutures. The stitches in the muscle layer were getting farther and farther apart. Thank God this was such a cooperative heifer. I tied the final knot and took a deep breath.

"Can you please take the lid off some more suture for me, Janet?" I pointed to the alcohol-filled container on the edge of the straw bale, then waited impatiently as the woman dried her hands before casually plucking the lid from the plastic container. "Just grab the string and pull it straight up."

She pulled up a few feet. I grabbed it below her hand and cut between our grips. I pulled up another three feet and whacked it off. Threading the heavy material into the eye of a cutting needle, I tied my first knot and proceeded upward with a series of interlocking stitches.

"Boy, there's sure lots of sewing." Mr. Schofer struggled to his feet and tottered to my elbow for a better view. I couldn't even respond. I hated that I couldn't be more animated with the man when this might be the only abdominal surgery he would ever see. Usually when I did surgery with a client for the first time, I loved talking about everything from the anatomy of the critter to the intricacies of the surgery itself. Today was not going to be my day for improving client-veterinarian relations!

My shirt was wet with sweat by the time I tied off the last of the skin sutures and threw my instruments in the box. I was in agony and determined to get out of there as quickly as possible. If I drove like a madman, there was still a remote chance of getting home with clean drawers.

With surgery box in hand, I made it to the first fence. Studying it with horrible apprehension, I realized that scaling this wall would be an impossible task—it may as well have been forty feet high! I searched for an alternative. "Does this gate open, Cliff?"

The quiet rancher looked surprised that I would ask such a foolish question. After all, he climbed over it twenty times a day. Why would anyone possibly want to open it? I stood rigidly with my legs clamped together as the confused man struggled to withdraw a one-inch pipe that slid into the adjoining gate to hold the two together. Not once in all the times I'd been coming to his farm had I ever asked for this barrier to be opened. The doors swung away from me and I took off like a shot.

"Thanks, Cliff!" I hollered over my shoulder. He smiled, brow furrowed, as I rushed by him. He was obviously having trouble putting his finger on why I was not my usual self. I could hear the structure rattle closed behind me—could feel the man's eyes on my back as I retreated down the alley. I could hear Lug whining as I scaled the final gate.

I did reach the car, and I did make it home with my dignity intact. At the time I was sure I was the only veterinarian in the world who had ever endured such an experience. I suspected, however, that was not the case. I'd never know for sure, though—it wasn't a popular topic of discussion at veterinary conferences.

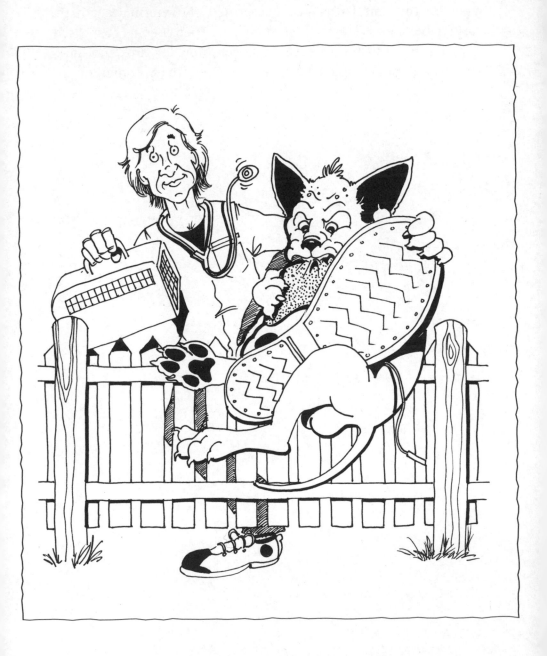

Dave and Goliath

The office was humming with conversation. Everyone sat patiently waiting for us to catch up. Doris was typing up the prescription label for Tiger Johnson's worm pills, and I had just finished vaccinating the Parkers' newly acquired cocker spaniel.

Sprite was the sweetest thing. At nine weeks old, he was a wriggling ball of yellow fluff with little pointed teeth. I was encouraging him to lick the final traces of Strongid T dewormer from a three-millilitre syringe when the telephone rang. Doris rolled her eyes at me.

"I'm done with Sprite," I said. "You finish up with the prescription and I'll take the call."

My harried receptionist returned her attention to the Underwood. She and I were at about the same skill level when it came to typing—two fingers and plenty of correction tape.

"Creston Veterinary Clinic," I answered.

"Hi, Dave…Harry Sommerfeld here. Got a little job for you. I've taken some dairy cattle on trade for hay. Is there any chance that I could get you to stop by to look after them? There's an old cow to have a peek at and six calves to castrate and dehorn."

"Shouldn't be a problem, Harry. When would you like to do them?"

"Could have some help here later this afternoon if you can make it."

I checked the daybook. Bill Merkley's name had been scrawled across the page for the last two hours of the afternoon but now had a line through it. He had scheduled a horse castration a couple of days before, but I cancelled it when I found out that the colt had not yet been vaccinated for tetanus. I'd backed it off until later in the month.

"How about three o'clock?"

"Sounds good to me," Harry replied. "Will you need anything special?"

"Shouldn't do. Are the horns already starting to develop? If they're still buds, we could do them with a caustic paste."

Doris hustled toward me. She thrust the little bottle of worm pills, a pen, and the vaccination certificate under my nose, indicating for me to hurry up.

"They're a pretty good size," Harry assured me.

"Mrs. Johnson wants to talk to you about her old dog, Shep," Doris whispered. "Don't take all day…Henrietta has Joey out in the car. She's bringing him in for a nail trim."

"We'll see you at three then, Harry."

I hung up the phone and got into the flow of the day. We raced from client to client until just before noon. When the last of the small animal appointments was finished, I headed up the stairs.

"I'm going to change my pants and slap together a sandwich, Doris."

"All right…looks like you better eat while you can. You have some horses to deworm in Wynndel at one."

I raced upstairs and hastily downed a peanut butter sandwich. I was stepping into my blue jeans when Doris called up the stairs.

"Dave! Can you take the phone?"

"Who is it?"

"Gabe Nugent. He has a problem with Sylvester."

"Great," I moaned. I traipsed to the upstairs phone, still pulling on my jeans. "Hello."

"Hi there, Doc. Sorry to bother ya now, but my Sylvester just got home 'n' he's a real mess."

"What seems to be the problem, Gabe?"

"Old bugger's bin scrappin' again. Ya know what he's like."

"Yeah, I do." I shook my head at the thought of the burly tom-cat with scar tissue like leather on either side of his neck. As lean as a cougar, he'd still weigh in close to fifteen pounds.

"He's bin gone the better part of a week this time—almost gave up on the old fart." Gabe's voice trailed off. There was a rattling of the phone as it landed on a countertop. "Goliath! Git to hell away from him before he hangs a lickin' on ya!"

I could just see the pesky chihuahua pestering the toughest cat in Erickson—that little mutt was one critter that knew absolutely no bounds. I waited for Gabe to come back to the phone.

"Sorry, Doc. Had to boot Goliath outside. Ya know how them two are. Goliath bugs the shit outta Silly…The ol' boy usually takes it, but this afternoon things might be different."

"So, what's the problem with Sylvester?" I had a tendency to get a bit impatient with Gabe—especially when he sounded as if he had been into the sauce. Today was no different.

"His face is all swoll up even worse than last time—remember what he was like? Right now he can't even open his eye. Got a big hunk o' fur missin' off his tail, too…Hate to leave him like that too long. Remember what happened when that hunk o' skin died off back o' his ear? He still don't grow hair back there."

"Sounds like we should look at him right away. How long do you think it'll take you to get him here?"

There was a long pause. "Ah, I think maybe ya better come 'n' git him, Doc…Got my licence suspended last week 'n' I'm not in very good shape today."

"Okay, Gabe, I'll come out. Where do you live?"

"Back Erickson Road…number 1532."

"Okay, I'll jump in the car right now."

I was about to hang up when Gabe started again. "I have to tell ya, Doc. Ya sure was right about Goliath. Never woulda thought he could do without all them teeth. Ya told me he could munch on dry dog food, but ya should see how he tackles his bones…Them gums are just like steel."

I chuckled at the thought of a toothless chihuahua munching away on a huge knucklebone.

"I'll see you in a bit then, Gabe."

Leaving Lug with Doris, I grabbed the biggest cat carrier we had and headed for the car. Gabe was quite the man. Prone to imbibing six or seven nights of the week, he was a character through and through. Although he seemed suspicious of almost every recommendation I had ever made to him, he usually went along with what I suggested and still called the office when he needed help.

He could have prevented most of his hassles by getting Goliath and Sylvester neutered. Both his pets were as feisty as he, and each carried far too much weight in his scrotum. I had drained an abscess for "Silly" not three months ago and had recommended that the old cat be neutered at the same time. Old Gabe had given me an incredulous look when I told him he was wasting an opportunity. He rolled his eyes.

"It'll keep him home and out of fights," I advised.

"Probably think it'd keep me home, too," the man asserted. "Nah—all three of us'll croak with our sacks full."

I drove down Erickson Road looking for 1532. I got to the 1400s and slowed down as I approached a row of four or five houses. I crept along, unable to find numbers on any of them. The next identified place was in the 1600s. Turning around, I idled back and pulled into a driveway on the west side of the road. A hundred feet up the lane, I stopped in front of the white stucco dwelling, dug out the cat carrier, and rang the doorbell. I had almost given up on an answer when I heard shuffling inside the house. The inner door opened hesitantly. An elderly woman stepped forward.

"Can I help you?" she asked, cautiously peering through the screen door.

"Yes. I'm looking for 1532—Gabe Nugent. He has a problem with his cat."

"That'd be next door." She pointed a gnarled, nicotine-stained finger to the little bungalow on the other side of a white picket fence.

"Thank you."

I was almost to the car when I hesitated. Why drive to Gabe's? It made more sense for me to detour across country rather than drive all the way around and up the long driveway next door. After all, the houses were not more than fifty feet apart.

I thought it somewhat strange that the woman stood on her doorstep watching as I strode up to the fence. I waved to her and ventured over, left leg first. A short fence like this was nothing to me. It was close to three feet high, but my legs measured a good thirty-seven inches when I stood flatfooted. I adjusted the crotch of my jeans when I got caught on a picket, and hefted my other leg up. Suddenly, I felt a jabbing pain at the back of my left leg. Withdrawing in shock, I retracted my limb. There, clinging tenaciously to my Achilles tendon, was Goliath, the toothless chihuahua.

"Let go, you little bugger!" I cried.

Reefing backwards, I shook my leg aggressively. Sharp picket ends drove deep into the crack of my arse and I recoiled. I tried swinging my other leg over, but the impaled denim kept me straddling the fence.

"Damn it, Goliath!"

I swung the cat carrier in an attempt to dislodge the mutt, but instead managed to deliver a sound whack to my ankle. Lifting my affected leg to the height of the top picket, I tried desperately to get hold of the miniature dynamo that clung to my foot as if his life depended on it. I grabbed his tail and reefed toward me. His beady eyes were filled with fury. I felt his jaw clamp down even tighter on my ankle.

"Aaaahhhhh!" The tenacious creature had me in a dither. I threw the cat carrier to the ground and grasped the cross rail of the fence. Flinging my right leg over, I pried my jeans free of the pickets. I swung my leg as if kicking a football, and Goliath flew through the air. He hit the ground and rolled end over end.

"Yip, yip yip! Yip, yip yip!"

I picked up the cat carrier, ready to give the dog a whack should he get adventurous once more. He barked ferociously, darting around just out of my reach.

"Goliath! Git in here!" Gabe hollered out the front door. "Sorry, Doc…Forgot I left him out there. Ya have to watch that little bugger…He's not above takin' a nip outta folks from time to time."

I glanced sheepishly over the fence at the helpful old lady who still stood in her doorway. The screen door was now fully open. Her face was alight with a huge smile. At least I had brought joy to someone's day. I walked into Gabe's cloistered living room.

"Yip, yip, yip…Yip, yip, yip…Yip, yip, yip!" Goliath danced around and around behind an overstuffed sofa. Every once in a while, he took a short run in my direction.

"Shut yer bloody trap, Goliath! Doc ain't here fer ya today. He's here fer Silly."

Hustling the dog into the adjacent bedroom, Gabe closed the door and separated us from the yapping chihuahua. I looked around the room in search of Sylvester. The blinds were down. The room was dark and the air smelled stale and musty. I stood for a few moments letting my eyes adjust to the change in light.

"Over here, Doc." Gabe motioned me to a wicker chair in the corner. The huge black and white cat lay stretched out on a floral seat cushion. "The ol' bugger sure took his licks this time… He must be slowin' down in his old age." Gabe clicked on the lamp that hung above the patient. "Can't see a bloody thing outta his eye."

I knelt down and ran my hand over the cat's body. Beneath his sleek hair coat was a multitude of scratches and scabs. He had indeed taken his share of the flack on this latest outing. I scratched my way forward and gently probed the area around his left eye.

The skin was taut and shiny from the pressure of the abscess beneath, but although there were a few scabs, there was no evidence that the skin was already dying off. I shook my head in awe as I ran my hands behind his ears. The skin there was as thick and callused as roughly tanned leather. No way was another cat likely to penetrate it. I ran my hand along Sylvester's body to the base of his tail, where the skin was torn open. Repair would be no big deal—he had lots of loose skin in that department.

"Well, Gabe, I'll take Silly with me and patch him up. He needs to have that abscess drained and the tear at the base of his tail stitched up. They'll both have tubes in them, and he may well have a hood on his head. You'll have to keep him at home for a bit."

"Shouldn't be a problem," Gabe mused. "He's had his toot fer now, and he'll hang around fer a bit expectin' me to spoil him."

"I don't suppose you want me to neuter him this time around?" I opened the cat carrier and lifted the huge critter off his cushion.

"Nah, not this time, Doc," Gabe muttered. "Poor old bugger's got enough on his plate."

"What did you do to yourself? You're limping." Doris watched me lug Sylvester in and plunk him on the table.

"You wouldn't believe it. That mutt of Nugent's got hold of my leg. It hurts like the dickens."

"That little chihuahua? You have to be kidding."

I gave Doris a look that put an immediate end to her banter, then opened the cat carrier and pried our reluctant patient from within. If the truth were known, although my Achilles tendon was indeed sore, it was the self-induced traumas that were causing the most discomfort. My ankle throbbed where I had whacked it with the carrier, and my groin was tender from the massage of the pickets.

"Oh my!" Doris exclaimed. "He doesn't look like a very happy camper."

"Another war wound…This critter will soon have more scar tissue than skin."

"Are we going to neuter him as well?"

"No way Gabe wants to even consider it. I think it would in some way detract from his own manhood."

"Humph!" Doris snorted. "Typical man."

By the time I had dealt with Silly's problems and dewormed the horse in Wynndel, the early afternoon had eroded. It was a beautiful day, and the drive from the north end of the valley to Lister gave me twenty minutes to enjoy the panoramic view of the rolling hills and surrounding mountains.

I had made sure that all of the materials I would need for the Sommerfeld call were in the vehicle before I left. Hoping that the animals were still young enough for its use, I had thrown in a bottle of caustic dehorning paste. If a farmer caught the calves early enough, the caustic could be applied to the buds to stop the horn growth. When applied properly, it handled the problematic procedure with far less brutality. If there was too much growth, I'd have to use gougers and accept the fact that there'd be a bit of blood.

Dehorning and castration of cattle were procedures that still bothered me. I hated causing unnecessary pain. Although we used some form of anesthesia whenever we cut into other species, with cattle it was expected that veterinarians would keep costs at a bare minimum. I followed procedure because it was required of me, but that didn't mean I liked it.

I passed the golf course on the way to Harry's. It seemed that half the businessmen in Creston were out there wandering around in the afternoon sun chopping holes in the turf. I wondered almost dreamily if I would ever get to the point where I'd be out there hacking along with them. Somehow, I doubted it.

I drove through the alfalfa fields of Lister, passed the school, and turned north at the next intersection. Instead of taking the main road that led to the picturesque community of Canyon, I proceeded straight ahead for an additional half mile. I pulled up to the drive of a farmhouse surrounded by trees and a quarter acre of lawn. Four men stood idly chatting in the carport. I recognized Harry and his brother, Hugo. The other two appeared to be Rune Anderson and Jim Moman. I wondered what they were all doing here. Ah, there was Harry's three-ton hay truck, all loaded and chained for a trip down the highway. The men must have just finished helping with the load. Harry hustled from the pack and approached as I pulled in.

"Hi, Dave. I'll maybe get you to have a quick look at the cow first. She's got this huge lump on her jaw, and I'm wondering if there's something I can do for her."

We strode through a well-manicured yard toward a collection of buildings north of the house. In a small enclosure newly constructed of rough-sawn lumber stood a black and white Holstein cow. Still munching a mouthful of hay, she lifted her head as we approached.

"How long has she been like that?" The lump protruded from the jaw on the left side of her face.

"I have no idea," Harry answered. "She's one of thirty head I took on trade for hay. Hughie, from up in Slocan, ran into a bit of trouble and sold out. Most of the decent cows went to other dairies...I took everything that he couldn't pawn off to anyone else."

I climbed over the rails and hopped to the ground next to the old cow. Scratching her on the tailhead, I quietly slipped a thermometer into her rectum. She turned her head to keep a wary eye on me. From where I was standing, I could see a conical gob of pink granulation tissue covered with white pus. I scratched my way along the spine and reached forward to feel the lump. It was rock-hard; the lesion felt like an extension of bone. I drifted back to remove the thermometer. Her temperature was normal.

"This looks like lump jaw, Harry. Most of what you see there," I said pointing to the lesion, "is a proliferation of bone." I climbed back out of the pen. "I'd contact the slaughterhouse and send her out rail-grade. Most of them will pass inspection so long as her temperature doesn't go up and there isn't any lymph node involvement."

"What causes it? It almost looks like cancer."

"A fungus called *Actinomyces bovis*. She probably got a barley awn or a piece of hay jammed up under her gum line, and the fungus gained entry. Once it gets into the bone, it's difficult to clear. Sodium iodide helps in the very early stages, but the only thing that ever seems to get rid of it is a drug used to treat tuberculosis in humans. You'd have to treat her twice a day for months, and very little of the bone you see here now would be remodelled."

"Well, I guess that settles that." Harry turned on his heel and headed for a clapboard structure that stood to the west of his machine shed. "I've got the calves in the chicken house over here…Been trying for years to get something to supplement the hay. I'm still not sure these cattle are a good idea. We raised some layers and tried peddling eggs around the Kootenays…said to hell with it after going to Kimberley with a load and bringing every one of them back. Did a bit better with broilers, but everyone seems to want them for nothing, too."

I nodded my head in sympathy. It was tough trying to make a good living with a small family farm these days.

"Do you think we can use the pinchers?" Harry asked. "I talked to some of the dairymen, and they mentioned just crimping the cord or putting on rubber rings."

"We may be able to do them with the burdizzo…That's the rig you're talking about for crushing the cord. I wouldn't use the rings on anything but newborns."

"I guess that rules out these fellas, then." Harry stopped at the shed and peered warily through the crack at the margin of the door. "Okay, guys!" He waved to the house and the other men gravitated in our direction. "We had a hell of a time getting them in here, and they're still probably more than a little worked up."

150

I opened the latch, but Harry cautioned me. "Be careful…if that big sucker gets out of there, we may never get him back."

I walked along the shed and peeked in a window that was at my eye level. I couldn't believe it—there peering back at me was a massive Holstein bull. He snorted at the sight of me, blowing snot through the open hole. My jaw dropped and I turned to stand face to face with the crew of hesitant hay farmers.

"I thought you said these were calves, Harry."

He smiled meekly. "Did you see the big one?"

"I hope so," I replied hesitantly. "Do you have some sort of a chute rigged up? How are we going to keep them still?"

"I was hoping you were going to tell us. I've been doing nothing but fencing trying to keep these guys in…Never had much to do with cattle before." Harry took off his glasses and polished them with the corner of his shirt. "That one big bugger is pretty handy with his horns. He's been nothing but trouble since we got him home."

I took a deep breath and headed for my car. This was going to be interesting. The words of Dr. Armstrong, my ambulatory instructor at the vet college, echoed through my mind: *Never let your client think that you know how to use a lariat. Better still, never let him know that you even have one—otherwise, you'll never have an animal confined and ready for you when you get there.*

I had no doubt at the time that he was right. The only problem was that he never did suggest what on earth to do when presented with six Holstein bulls rampaging around in a chicken house. At least I could forget about dragging the caustic paste over there. I dug through my kit box for my largest set of gougers, then cut off a four-foot section of embryotomy wire. Hell, the gouger I had wouldn't begin to touch the horns of the critter that I had seen. This was going to be the rodeo to end all rodeos.

"Exactly how did you plan on controlling these critters, Harry?" I was hoping he had something magical up his sleeve. He gave me a blank look in return. "Is there anything to tie them to

151

in there?" I looked wistfully through the crack in the door.

Harry thought for a moment before he shook his head. "Nothing that would hold them."

"Maybe I better get in there and get a feel for what we're up against." I removed the two-by-six that was propped under the doorknob and opened the door a crack.

"Don't show that big brute too much air, or he'll be through in a flash." Harry waited as I slipped through the narrow opening, then slammed it behind me.

I scanned the small space as my eyes grew accustomed to the gloom. Four black and white calves were lined up in a row hiding their heads from me. All I could see were their rumps. Thank God they weren't all the size of the first one. I looked in his direction. He stood facing me next to another critter that was almost as big. Both watched me attentively. I worked my way around the room in the semi-darkness trying to envision some way of controlling these beasts while I magically deprived them of their horns and testicles. Harry was right—there was nothing here to tie them to. I knocked on the inside of the door, hoping that someone was still within earshot.

"Hello! Harry?"

I heard the prop being removed. The door opened a crack and I squeezed through.

"We need to rig up something to tie them to. Better get a hammer and some spikes."

Harry took off in the direction of his carport.

I smiled at the grey-haired fellow who stood nervously scratching at the eczema on the back of his hand. "You've got a crew of reluctant cowboys here, Dave," he said.

"You're taking the afternoon off for a bit of excitement, I see."

"Guess you could say that."

I had met Rune Anderson through Gordon Veitch and bumped into him frequently in the milk parlours of the local dairymen. He was one of the most respected electricians in the area, and the

152

farmers were always singing his praise. I had passed his farm on the way over here. He had a hundred acres of alfalfa out on the main drag and lived in a nicely finished home right across from the school.

"We had the devil of a time even getting them in there. As you can see, Harry's not exactly set up for cattle...I think right about now he's wishing he had stuck with the chickens."

I laughed out loud. "I have to be honest with you—I'm sort of wishing he had, too. How did you get involved with this adventure?"

"Not exactly sure, but we're all in the Lister Co-op together. Harry trucks our hay and we try to help each other out."

"This would sure be a lot easier if he had a squeeze, or at least a chute. As it is, there's not a thing to tie them to. We have to get in there and nail something to the wall as a sort of anchor."

Harry returned with an armload of two-by-six scraps and some four-inch spikes. Within a few minutes, we had a tie structure banged together on the nearest corner.

"I'm not sure it'll hold those big buggers," I said, "so maybe we better start small."

While Harry headed to the house for a bucket of water, the boys guarded the door. I made a loop with my lariat and took a few reluctant steps into the building. The two bigger bulls stood facing me, raising and lowering their huge heads as they evaluated my progress. The four smaller animals stuck together, their heads in a corner, their butts toward me. I worked my way between the wall and the closest critter, widening my loop as I inched along. I got the rope around his horns and slipped it over his head. He shifted slightly, lowering his head in an attempt to get away from me. I formed a half hitch, slipped it over his nose, and tightened it.

"Okay, guys. Someone take the rope."

Rune and Jim Moman crept in to join the action, and I threw them the end of the lariat.

153

"Get it around our anchor and reel him in."

I tapped the bull on the nose and backed him from the corner. He twirled and lowered his head. Pushing his buddies in front of him, he headed away from me.

"Yah! Get back!" Jim roared as the four critters charged directly toward the two men. "Damn! Get off my foot!"

The free bulls fought their way through the entanglement of rope and human bodies to join their larger counterparts at the other end of the chicken house. Our first hapless victim, now alone, yanked on the halter that encircled his head. Twisting from side to side, he leaned back on all fours and bellowed.

"Cinch him tighter, guys!" I hollered. "Bring him right up to the corner."

Jim gave the critter a whack on the hip, and as the animal charged forward, Rune took up the slack. I slipped outside to grab my dehorners. As much as I hated the inhumanity of this procedure, it was time to get on with it. As I approached, the critter was still leaning back against the rope in hopes of freeing himself. I slipped the mouth of the gougers over the horn by the wall and lunged. The blades of the dehorners sliced through the bone with a sickening crunch. The critter emitted a plaintive bawl. I flipped the horn to the barn floor and repeated the procedure on the opposite side. Blood sprayed from the pair of craters in the bull's head. Pulling the container of blood stopper from my pocket, I dusted the wounds.

"Have you got the water ready, Harry? We need you."

Rune and Jim stood on either side of the animal as I checked his testicles. They were both there and very well developed.

"Are you going to just crimp the cords?" Harry asked.

"I could, but wouldn't if they were my animals. When you crimp them, you just cut off the blood supply to the testicle. The nut tends to shrivel up, but sometimes it's tough for a buyer to be sure they've been done. If he has any doubt, he won't give you the same price for them."

Harry passed me the bucket of water, and I grabbed the soap container that bobbed within it. I looked directly at Rune and Jim to impress my next point.

"You guys have to be careful to pay attention when you're holding his tail. Hold it just like this." I lifted the tail straight over the animal's back and pushed it firmly ahead. "If you don't keep enough pressure on it, or don't hold it straight ahead, he'll kick me. My day already started off a bit rough—I don't want to end it with a kick."

Both men stared at me and at the tail. Jim smiled at Rune, then grabbed hold.

"A little lower," I instructed, "and straight ahead."

I squatted behind the animal and washed my hands. Opening the castration pack, I slipped a blade onto the scalpel handle and dropped it into the soapy water. Next, I splashed water on the scrotum and slathered it with soap. Cutting it the entire length, I maneuvered my finger around the tunic that enclosed the testicle and worked it free. The bull extended both legs as I pushed upward to leave the testicle dangling. I withdrew the stainless steel emasculators from the pack at my feet, opened them, and slipped them over the cord. Jim winced as the handles closed and steel crunched through the tissue. He straightened himself as if feeling sympathy pains.

"Oh, my God—that sound."

I repeated the procedure on the opposite side, then stood back to make sure there was no bleeding. I had enough residual discomfort from my earlier encounter with the picket fence to be more than a little sympathetic.

"Okay, guys...one down."

I released the steer. He wandered off to the far corner and stood dejectedly by himself. His ears drooped; blood trickled slowly down both sides of his head.

After half an hour of thrashing around, almost everyone was nursing a sore spot or two. With twenty-four sets of hooves in such confined quarters, it was almost impossible to avoid getting tromped on. The first three small animals went fairly well, but the fourth gave us a real run for our money.

We pounded around that shed for the better part of twenty minutes trying to catch him. The air was heavy with dust and dander from the poultry litter, and feathers floated everywhere. I was hot on the critter's tail and sure that I had him this time. He was charging straight toward Rune when I threw my loop. The calf stopped on a dime, twirled in the opposite direction, and once more ducked my lariat. The problem was that he pivoted on Rune's toes. The poor man let out a holler, cursed in pain, and limped toward the door. I continued my pursuit for two more steps, then hesitated. I was face to face with the big black bull.

Lowering his head at me, he was ready to stand his ground. The look in his large brown eyes brought me up short. The small blotch of white on his massive forehead was covered with blood from the other critters. It was obvious that his patience with our game of round-and-round-the-chicken-coop had run thin. He snorted, then raised and lowered his head once more. Slowly and deliberately, he pawed at the floor.

"Time for a coffee break!" I yelled.

Rune and Jim quickly agreed, and before the bull threw any more chicken manure and feathers into the air, we vacated the building.

"Things are getting a bit tense in there," I muttered to Harry. "I think it's time to do that big boy and get him out of there. Holstein bulls are not noted for their tolerance…We've all but worn out our welcome with him."

"I hope that tie in the corner will hold him," said Rune.

"That makes two of us. He must weigh close to fifteen hundred pounds."

I peeked through the crack in the door. The black bull's menacing eyes glared back at me. He definitely needed time to cool off. We retreated to the carport.

"Is the coffee ready, Elaine?" asked Harry.

His wife called from the kitchen. "It will be in just a minute! I wasn't expecting you to finish so quickly."

We all laughed at once and Harry replied, "Neither were we."

At this point in my career, it was all I could do to get a cup of coffee down. This particular farm visit may well have been the beginning of my appreciation for the beverage. The conversation over the break was focused almost completely on how to deal with the spirited black rebel. There was no reason we should have been surprised that the animal would be hard to handle. Dairy bulls were notorious for their feisty attitude, and many a careless farmer had paid the price for not giving them their due respect.

"We definitely need to thin out the population in there," I chimed. "Maybe we can get a rope on that big sucker and let the ones we've finished go."

"I don't know," Harry said. "We had a devil of a time getting them in there to start with. I'd sure hate to lose one and not get him done."

I wandered back to the chicken coop while the boys were savouring the last few sips of coffee in the safety of the carport. Approaching the west side of the shed, I sneaked up to the first window. The calves were all close to the other end. The ones that had already been handled stood with their heads stuck in the corner while the others milled about near the door. The big bull lowered and raised his head, huffing and snorting into the crack at the side of the door, determined to escape from the enclosure.

"Any ideas?" Harry was standing behind me with Jim at his side. The moment the bull heard the man's voice, he charged the length of the fifty-foot shed. Stopping short of the wall, he shook his enormous head and let out a long savage bellow.

"Not really...and it appears that the coffee break has done little to settle his nerves."

As if to emphasize my statement, the critter thrust his head at the window. Throwing snot in all directions, he snorted again and again. I ran for my lariat. "Maybe I can get him through the window."

The bull backed off a step as I fiddled with the loop on the rope, trying to make it large enough to go over his horns.

"Watch he doesn't get your arm caught between his horn and the wall," Harry cautioned.

Jim shook his head in disgust. "By God, baling hay's looking better by the minute."

At this moment, Elaine joined the men to observe the goings-on. She laughed at Jim's joke, well aware of the trials of farming with big animals.

I threw the rope. Deflected by a horn, it settled ineffectually over the bull's forehead. The animal charged after my retreating arm. His horns struck the wall with a thundering crash, and the board beneath the window splintered. The rope slipped off the moment I tried to tighten it.

"That son of a bitch has been a problem since he got off the truck," Harry complained. "With those long legs and that set of horns, there's not a fence on the place he can't take out if he sets his mind to it."

I walked the length of the building, trying to come up with some sort of strategy. There was not much doubt that we were going to have to rope him through a window. It would be suicide to get in there with him again. There were a few narrow windows along the length of the building. Although they had once been glassed, none of them remained intact, but being more than five feet from the ground, they made for awkward throwing. I length-ened my noose and fooled with the loop until it stayed in a nice circle.

"You guys see if you can keep his attention over there."

Jim waved his hand through the window and banged on the shiplap wall of the building. The bull lowered his head and pawed at the floor. Propping a rickety apple box under the window, I mounted it and teetered back and forth. I lunged and managed to get the rope over one of the bull's horns. He reefed back and struggled to free himself.

"You got him!" someone shouted.

The bull charged backwards like a freight train. *Got him, indeed!* The rope sizzled through my hands as I helplessly tried to impede him. With a resounding crash, he collided with the opposite wall.

"Everyone grab the rope!"

As the bull struggled against the tether, everyone dove to help. With all hands pulling, the tug-of-war was on—the Lister Hay Producers versus the Feisty Slocan Bull. Ever so slowly the men began to dominate, and more and more of the rope appeared outside the building.

"Keep up the good work, you guys!"

I abandoned them, grabbed another rope, and ran around the shed to the far door. Removing the props that held it shut, I shooed the other critters to the opposite side and entered. I warily approached our reluctant patient. With all four feet planted, the bull leaned back against the rope and emitted a low-pitched grumbling from deep within his throat. Still focusing on resisting the force that dragged him toward the window, he stood firm as I worked the other rope over his horn and around his nose. I ran it around the tie we had used for the other bulls and began to pull.

"Can I have someone to help me here?"

Within a few seconds, Jim appeared at the door and cautiously worked his way over to me. With both of us leaning into the rope, the beast slowly started to give up ground. Still grumbling, he stood with feet planted, occasionally shaking his head. Taking a half hitch around the wall tie so that Jim could control him by himself, I positioned myself behind the bull, leaned on his hips, and cranked on his tail. Half step by half step, the critter moved closer and closer to the corner.

"Tie onto something out there and throw in the end of that big cotton rope!" I hollered.

The rope flew through the window to land in coils at my feet. I worked it under the bull's throat and along his side and threw it out the next window.

"Pull him tight to the wall!"

Holding the rope against the animal's side, I leaned into him. The critter was soon right where I wanted him.

"Steady as she goes! Pass me the water through the window." With all other hands in active duty, Elaine pitched in. She lifted the bucket with the soap and instruments, and I retrieved it.

"I guess this is it, Jim...Tie him off there and we'll get on with the show."

"Do you think it'll hold him?"

"We'll soon find out."

I cranked the bull's tail straight over his back and motioned for Jim to take over my position.

"Just remember the only thing that stands between me and that bull kicking me is you keeping pressure on the tail straight ahead. I don't know why it works, but it does when it's done properly." I looked Jim right in the eye. "I don't need to tell you how hard this big sucker could kick me."

I started scrubbing the set of prodigious testicles while my assistant leaned into the bull and struggled with the ponderous tail. I finished my scrub and held the testicles firmly to the end of the sac. As the scalpel cut through the scrotum, sweat beaded on Jim's forehead. His right arm trembled. The bull straightened both hind legs as I made first one incision, then the other. I worked both testicles free and applied the emasculator. The bull gave a pathetic little blat...Jim's face twitched reflexively at the sound of the crunch.

"One down."

I left the device in place for three minutes, allowing sufficient time to assure good stasis of blood flow. By the time I removed the emasculator and reapplied it to the opposite side, sweat flowed freely down Jim's face. I stood up and stretched my back.

"Can I let him go now?" Jim's request sounded more like a plea.

"Just two more minutes."

I waited patiently for the time to expire, then released the emasculators. The moment I could see that there was no hemorrhage, I signalled for Jim to let him go. He almost looked disappointed when the critter just stood there. I tied the handles onto a section of embryotomy wire and moved to his head. Looping the wire around the immense horn, I leaned back and began sawing. As the wire bit deeply into the horn, the acrid smell of smoke assailed us. Jim watched, dumbfounded as the wire got closer and closer to the forward edge. Within another dozen strokes, the horn separated from the creature's head and fell to the ground.

"My God, if that don't look better," I heard from the other side of the wall.

I huffed my way through the other horn, putting all my effort into keeping the wire smoking and getting the job done as quickly as possible. By the time the second horn fell to the ground, my shoulders and arms literally burned from exertion, and sweat poured off my face. I leaned my butt against the shed wall...Only two more to go.

With the other critters herded to the far corner, I vaccinated the big fellow and let him go. He walked resolutely toward the open door and Harry let him pass. Releasing the other animals went smoothly, and for some reason, working through the remaining two was a cakewalk.

By the time we were finished, however, every member of the crew was aware that he'd had a workout. Each man was plastered with enough blood and "green gold" to prove that he was a bona fide cowboy. I kept wanting to razz Jim about the chicken feathers embedded in his curly blond hair, but thought better of it.

"Boy, I'll tell you, Dave," he said as we were walking back to the house, "you've given me a new appreciation for hay farming."

"Glad to help, Jim, glad to help."

It seemed that each of us, save Harry's wife, moved with some sort of a limp. Poor Rune was unquestionably the worst off—I'd have been surprised if his toes weren't broken. I'd say I faired a close second with Harry. I'm not exactly sure how he got his injury, but I was damned if I was going to tell them how I got mine. I was hoping none of them ever talked to the old girl who lived next door to Gabe.

The Trials of Mrs. Beale

I was sure from the woman's directions that I had found the right place. It was the only house at the end of the meandering dirt road, and there sat the battered old green Ford pickup—just as she had described it. I was curious to meet her, to see the person that went with the timid voice on the other end of the phone. After two extended chats, I had finally convinced her that it was in her best interest to have her cow examined. Educated guesses were often worth little more than what one paid for them.

I walked through patches of weeds up the rickety landing and knocked on the plywood-covered door. There was shuffling inside—a murmur of children's voices. The door opened a crack and a tall, wispy woman peered nervously up at me. Her face was thin, almost gaunt. Adjusting her wire-rimmed glasses, she squeezed the bridge of black tape that bonded the two halves of the frame together.

"Mrs. Beale? I'm Dr. Perrin."

"Hello." Positioning her body to prevent me from seeing into the room behind her, she whispered, "I'll be right out." She closed the door.

I wandered toward the rusting relic in the driveway and gazed about the yard. Positioned in the centre of a large grove of trees, the house looked as if it had been dragged into place on skids and dumped when the mover could advance no further. It perched precariously on wooden blocks that supported the corners. Other than a few trees that had been sacrificed for the structure, no effort had been made to position the house for a view or to allow it even

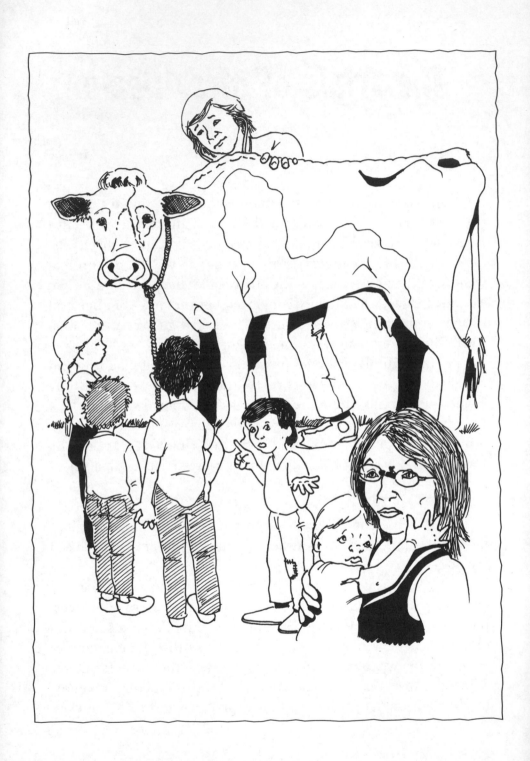

the faintest peek at the sun. I glanced around for evidence of a garden, but the ground was undisturbed.

A Doberman-cross bitch with long, stretched nipples slunk from beneath the far side of the building and rattled her way to the end of a heavy metal chain. I hadn't even noticed her on my first approach to the house, and she seemed determined to distance herself from me as much as possible.

The front door squeaked open, and Mrs. Beale exited the house with a child in her arms. Held firmly to his mother's breast, with his arms around her neck, the boy buried his face in her shoulder. As I watched, four others swarmed from the house to surround her, each a head shorter than the next and all dressed in well-worn clothing. A few knees and elbows protruded from ragged holes.

Gently nudging a toddler to one side, Mrs. Beale balanced precariously on one leg and slipped her foot into a rubber boot. She repeated the performance with the other foot, then descended the stairs with her entourage close behind her.

"The cow's over this way," she said, her voice as hollow as her cheeks.

Like a flock of quail, they led me down a well-defined path into the bush. The children stayed so close to their mother that I was sure she'd trip. As I followed her, I wondered if there was yet another Beale already on the way. The poor woman had obviously not gotten into the rhythm of birth control, while her husband had no intention of missing a beat.

"She's in there." The dishevelled convoy stopped and the woman pointed into the trees. "I tried to get Myron to call you last week, but he said she's just constipated."

I peered in the direction that Mrs. Beale pointed. There on the ground behind a massive fir tree was a motionless black and white mound.

"Myron was in to Sunset Seed to buy mineral oil yesterday," she went on. "He was gonna drench her, but it was after dark when he got home… and I don't think he got around to it."

The haggard woman struggled to adjust the child's weight on her hip as the others clung to her. They eyed me warily. Pushing her sagging glasses back up the sharp bridge of her nose, she again applied pressure to the black tape.

"My sister came by this morning with a nice bale of alfalfa hay. We tried and tried to tempt the cow but couldn't get her to take even a mouthful…I'm kinda worried we left her too long."

I picked my way through a clump of stunted alders and stopped a few paces from the animal. Lying with her head resting on her hind leg, the creature was totally uninterested in my approach. Her eyes were closed; her muzzle was dry and crusted with fir needles. A ponderous logging chain hung from her neck, seeming to weight her head to the ground. I grabbed the constraint and hefted it forward up the cow's neck. A deep impression remained where it had rested—the underlying area was rubbed hairless and flies crawled over a raw spot at the crown of her poll. A flake of prime green alfalfa hay lay untouched on the ground under her jaw.

"I was hoping that hay'd get her eating, but…" Mrs. Beale's voice faded.

"What else have you been feeding her?" I ran my hand over the cow's prominent ribs.

"We got some grassy hay from Myron's brother, and I've been tethering her out here."

I looked about me in search of a blade of grass, and then turned my attention back to the cow. She lay in a rather unusual position with her shoulders slightly abducted from her body. Although her breathing was slow and regular, each exhalation was punctuated with a low grunt.

"Have you been giving her grain at all?"

The family moved nearer to me, and the older boy, who appeared to be seven or eight, ventured a few steps closer than his mother. The woman shook her head.

166

"Has she been up this morning?" Again the woman shook her head.

I fished my thermometer from my coveralls and unscrewed the top. I shook down the mercury, spit on my hand, and rotated the instrument in the saliva for lubrication. I struggled to insert it into the cow's rectum. The mucous membranes were dry, and the device entered only grudgingly.

"What has her milk been like?" I asked.

"I only got enough to cover the bottom of the bucket last night," Mrs. Beale sighed. "When we got her back in April she was filling it right to the brim."

"Has the milk been clear…No signs of little flakes or cheesy lumps?"

"Nothing on the tea towel when I strain it."

I palpated the udder. Its texture felt good—no indication of the lumps of scar tissue that usually followed the ravages of a mammary infection. I knelt by the cow's head and lifted it with the pressure of my hand under her jaw. Her eyes opened but she stared vacantly past me. I explored the back of her mouth. A few stalks of the alfalfa hay still stuck to her tongue.

Moving back, I dug my knees into her side. "Get up, girl! Come on, get up!"

The animal stirred and grudgingly struggled against the logging chain until she stood with her head barely a foot from the ground, her elbows drawn away from her body. She grunted dramatically with each breath as if every movement of her rib cage caused pain.

Leaning against the cow's side, I used my stethoscope to listen to the sound of air flowing in and out of her lungs. I was trying to detect the gurgling of fluid in the airway—some indication of active pneumonia.

All I could hear was the deep, throaty vibration of air being forced through her closed glottis. Moving further down on her left side, I listened to her racing heart. I closed my eyes, intent on drowning out all outside input. Waiting for the sloshing sounds that indicate an infectious pericarditis, I switched to the right side and held my breath. I heard only the rapid, sharp contractions of the heart.

I grasped the cow's lumbar vertebrae and clamped down firmly with my hand. The cow depressed her withers, held her breath, and crouched in that position like an oversize marionette. Finally, she straightened and gave a deep-throated, painful moan. *Oh man, that hurt.*

"What in the hell is going on here?"

I turned with a start and pulled the stethoscope from my ears. Stumbling down the trail was Myron Beale. Mrs. Beale passed the toddler to her oldest son, and the children immediately shifted ten feet away from their mother.

"Diane, you stupid bitch…I told you I wasn't gonna waste money on a vet! What in the hell didn't you understand in that?"

"Well…I thought we should try. Maybe he can help—"

Her words stopped short. Towering over his wife, the man raised his right arm. Mrs. Beale cowered.

"Mr. Beale!" I roared. "Don't!"

The man lowered his arm and glared in my direction. His wife still stood half-crouched with her hands over her head. I closed the distance between us.

"We need the cow, Myron," she pleaded. "You know we need the milk."

Mr. Beale's scowl remained unchanged. He stared at me, obviously sizing up his chances, his green eyes squinting disdain. In his late thirties, Myron was an imposing man. Although he sported a well-earned beer gut, he was husky and not much shorter than I. My heart was pounding as I waited for him to make a move. Breathing heavily, he swayed back and forth. I stood close enough that the smell of stale beer and body odour was almost overpowering.

Mrs. Beale took advantage of the staring match to back away

168

toward her children. "We need the cow, Myron," she repeated.

The man's gaze broke from mine and drifted to the animal that stood hunched behind me.

"Need! Need! Need! Goddamnit, all you do is need!"

Without another glance at me, he wheeled around, stumbled over a root, and sprawled flat on the ground. There was a moment as he lay in the dirt that Mrs. Beale and I just watched him. Then picking himself up, he sneered at his wife and retreated down the path.

"Useless woman!" he hollered over his shoulder. "All you ever do is need!"

Mrs. Beale avoided my gaze. Wanting to spare her embarrassment, I returned to the cow and pretended to listen through the stethoscope, even though I knew there was nothing more to hear. But my hands trembled from the adrenaline rush and my mind raced.

Almost as an afterthought, I remembered the thermometer. I checked it and found the cow's temperature was 40.8 Celsius—two degrees above normal.

Calmer now, I turned around to face Mrs. Beale. She stared into the distance, seemingly lost, then met my eyes.

"I'm pretty sure I know what's wrong here...Your cow's got hardware."

The woman took a step in my direction, and her entourage moved with her. "Hardware?"

"It's slang. Means she swallowed...well...hardware."

"Oh." Mrs. Beale looked puzzled, still unsure she was getting my meaning.

"Cattle aren't very selective in their eating habits, and they end up downing the strangest things. The most dangerous are pieces of sharp wire and, of course, nails."

"She would really swallow something like that?"

I nodded.

"You know, I found some stuff in that hay Myron got from his brother. Some bits of barbed wire. But I never thought she'd eat any of it."

"Well, I'm betting she did."

"Oh no-o-o…I really do need the milk for the kids…" It was a question more than a statement, asking what I could do to help.

"I'll do what I can for her, but you have to realize the damage may not be reversible. Even if she does recover, with the condition she's in, she may never do much for milk until her next lactation."

Mrs. Beale's lower lip trembled. Tears welled and she shifted her son to try and wipe them away. As she removed her glasses, they separated, and one of the halves fell to the ground. I picked it up and handed it to her.

"I'll be right back."

I strode down the trail to my car, wondering how the woman could ever dig her way out of this despair. I doubted there was much food in that shack of a house, and I knew how much this family depended on this cow for milk. What a way to live. What a way to raise your children.

I fumbled through the stuff in the car, without much thought to what I was looking for. I stopped and took a deep breath, realizing that I was seething with rage. It was as if some vagrant anger had found a home—I wasn't sure where it came from or where it was directed.

Maybe I was angry with Mrs. Beale. She seemed so helpless—so willing to accept her lot in life. Or maybe I was angry at Mr. Beale, knowing that he'd hit her again—if not today, then soon. But I was angry with myself, too, because I would just walk away from this family and their situation. I was just a vet. After administering the cow's medications, I would be gone, leaving this woman and her children to whatever fate awaited them.

By the time I returned, Mrs. Beale had composed herself. She and the children stood in front of the cow, and she was offering it a handful of hay.

"We're going to give her antibiotics and hope that will wall off the infection in her tummy," I said. "For forty-eight hours after the last injection, the milk won't be fit for the children."

I held a sixteen-gauge needle in my fingertips so Mrs. Beale could observe. "I want you to hold it like this…Slap her like so." I hit the cow's rump gently a few times with the back of my hand. "Then drive it in."

I flipped my hand and drove the needle to the hub in the cow's rear end. "Leave it for a bit, make sure no blood runs out, then hook on the syringe and give the injection."

"What happens if blood does come out?" Mrs. Beale squinted through the one glass that balanced over her right eye.

"That means you hit a vessel. Pull out the needle and start again."

I connected the syringe and slowly injected the penicillin. The children watched attentively, then all looked to their mother when I pulled out the needle and massaged the injection site.

"Do you see this?"

I showed the children a three-inch round piece of gleaming metal, and then stuffed it into my pocket. When I pulled it out, my entire ring of keys dangled from it.

"This is a powerful magnet," I said. "What we're hoping is that it will grab hold of the wire or nail that's causing the problem and drag it back into your cow's first stomach. It won't cause trouble there."

All eyes watched in fascination as I dropped the magnet into a balling-gun and moved around to the front end of the cow. Grasping her upper jaw, I worked the long, cylindrical apparatus into her mouth and pushed the plunger. I withdrew the device and showed the kids that the magnet was gone.

"One more piece of metal in your cow's tummy."

The older boy smiled and looked up at his mother.

"How much will all this cost?" Mrs. Beale asked tentatively.

"You don't worry about that. This one's on me."

After I explained that the cow should be force-fed a solution of propylene glycol to give her energy, I demonstrated the procedure by forcing the liquid down her throat. The task required some strength, because even in its weakened state the cow was resisting. I wondered how in the world this frail woman would manage by herself.

Hell, for that matter, how could she handle any of this on her own? Like her wretched animal, Mrs. Beale was chained to her circumstances, prepared to swallow whatever was being fed to her.

I gathered my equipment together, wondering why I felt so disturbed by this pair. Was it because they seemed so helpless, or was it because my own existence was not much better as I ran from one disaster to the next, apparently unable or unwilling to take control?

As I headed back to the car, the woman and her children were wandering about the woods pulling a few blades of grass here and a dandelion there. The cow would at least have one good mouthful of feed should she decide to eat again. I drove from the place, wondering if there was any hope for Mrs. Beale or her hardware cow. At the moment, the prognosis for both of them seemed rather dismal.

Verna's Paternity Suit

My eyelids fluttered momentarily. Clamping them tightly together, I struggled to bar the bright rays of light that already streamed in my bedroom window. A transport truck rattled over the pothole in the pavement in front of the clinic and roared toward Cranbrook. I gently lifted Lug's head from my shoulder to glance at my watch. Six-fifteen—no way was I ready to give up on sleep yet. How could a relaxation-deprived vet not take advantage of a peaceful Sunday morning? The realization hit that the telephone hadn't rung once since noon yesterday.

Lug sighed deeply and rolled over on his back, giving no indication that I had interrupted his slumber. I strained to keep my eyes closed, hoping to drift off once more. Concentrating on the sound of the German shepherd's deep, relaxed breathing, I wished that I could learn his technique for letting go. Five long minutes later I admitted defeat and surrendered to a barrage of peripheral inputs. The bright light insistently pried its way through my lids, my bladder nagged to be emptied, my ear pleaded for scratching I took a deep breath, opened my eyes, and stretched. "Time to get up, boy."

Unceremoniously assisting Lug from the bed, I swung my feet to the floor. The big mutt stretched, arched his back, then presented his head to my lap in search of the ear rub that he'd grown to live for.

Time was flying of late. It seemed like only yesterday that I'd been venturing into darkness for calvings at seven and eight in the morning. Back in the early spring, it was gloomy by the time we

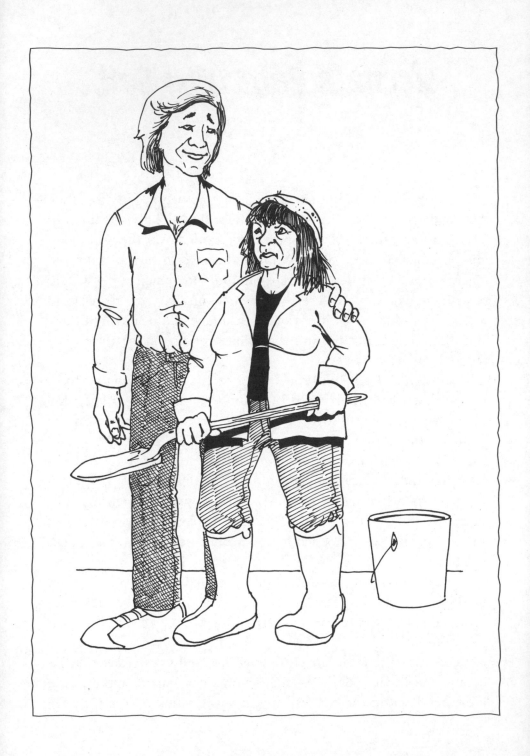

closed shop at five-thirty. Now it was light by four-thirty a.m. and still not dark by ten at night. These fine June days were primed to determine how much a man could pack into them.

Would I ever learn to manage the fleeting moment? I found it hard to believe that another birthday had come and gone. Twenty-eight years old…Pretty soon I'd be stumbling over the big three-zero.

The way the years were accumulating, it was time to stop wishing my life away. Right now, I was like a little kid waiting for summer break. June couldn't go fast enough. July was going to be a special month—one I was anxious to get on with. Not only would Cory be here to start work, but Brian would be back. I had called Ken Blair at the social services office the day before. He'd been in communication with Brian's caseworker in Taber, and it sounded like everything was on track. Martha had jumped through all the administrative hoops, and barring a veto from head office, he would be here in mid-July. The boy and I and Lug could spend a lot more time getting things done around the farm, and we'd damn soon be checking out new fishing holes.

Within the hour, I had set up a new IV bag, and fluids continued to drip into old Jeb's vein. I had already given him his injection of antibiotics. Except for a cat and another dog that were boarding, the rotund poodle was the only hospitalized patient. I carefully checked the blankets in his kennel for signs of vomitus and smiled to find them clean. It appeared that my fat little friend had finally stopped vomiting! This morning there was even a faint twitch of his tail as I plucked him from the kennel and carried him outside. Today he was looking as if he just might want to live.

I had been feeling so sorry for him. He had presented two days earlier with a rigid posture and long ropes of drool that hung from his jowls. His doting owner, Norm, was at his wit's end as he watched his buddy throw up again and again. He knew Jeb was in dire straits when he saw the revulsion the little mutt had for even his favourite treat. Normally, a spoonful of liver sausage would have had the overgrown poodle doing cartwheels.

This was the third time that a bout of pancreatitis had caused my patient to be presented for treatment. I hoped that this episode had been frightful enough to get through to Norm. He insisted on feeding the dog from the table, even though I'd been nagging that Jeb should get nothing other than unadulterated dry dog food.

"But he just sits there with this hungry look!" was Norm's favourite response. "How can I possibly enjoy my own dinner with him perched on his chair next to me staring with those big brown eyes?"

My suggestion that the dog be put outside or locked in another room while Norm ate only earned me a look of total incredulity. The idea was so without merit that the portly man could not even consider it. Instead, he went on defending his actions. "But I've really worked to cut down on the fat in his diet."

"What did you feed him the night before this episode?" I pursued.

Norman responded hesitantly. He shifted his feet and placed one loafer on top of the other as he leaned back against the wall. He took his eyes off the face of his woebegone pet for just a moment and stared into the waiting room. His voice dropped almost to a whisper. "A pork chop…"

"A pork chop?"

"I trimmed most of the fat off," Norm answered defensively. His voice trailed off. "I guess that wasn't the best, was it?" His forehead was creased and his blue-green eyes emitted despair. "I love pork chops…We haven't been having them lately because of Jeb. I'm sorry…I guess I'll have to give them up completely."

Norm was still not capable of entertaining the thought that he and his friend could eat separately. I knew from past conversations that the two ate every meal together seated side by side at the kitchen table. I could just picture that spoiled mutt sitting in his highchair, waiting for Norm to finish cutting up his pork chop. I smiled at the image of the man and his dog with a bowl of kibble in front of each of them. I wondered if Norm would consider changing his own diet to Purina Dog Chow.

We arrived at the farm before nine o'clock. Lug tore off in front of me as I walked from the hay shed to the clearing in my forest. How he loved the freedom of this place. How he treasured his position at the top of the animal hierarchy. Before taking a dozen steps, he had picked up a three-foot-long pine branch and begun his ritual. Howling as if in agony, he chased back and forth in front of a cow-calf pair until he sent them scattering.

"Get over here, you big goof!"

Coming almost close enough for me to reach the stick, he howled again and chomped repeatedly on the ill-fated wood. As I stooped to grab it, he took off ahead of me, still wailing and growling for all he was worth.

I made several trips back and forth for fence posts before I started digging. Many of the old cedar posts that George Sikora, the original owner, had put in were rotten at ground level, and one by one, they were giving out. As I watched, a Hereford cow pressed her twelve hundred pounds against the strands of the barbed-wire fence in search of a mouthful of grass on the other side. The wires creaked and groaned as she stretched yet farther afield for that one blade she couldn't quite reach.

"Hey, you old bat! No wonder I can't keep a fence up here."

I shooed her away. The old saying that good fences made good neighbours certainly applied here. The last thing I needed was for this section of wire to fail. My neighbour, Verna, and I had already had enough conflict to last me for this lifetime. It had been months since we had exchanged scowls, and I think she was finally getting used to the idea that I was here to stay. I didn't want anything to upset the apple cart.

Soon I had two of the green treated posts planted and the dirt tamped firmly around them. I put the last staple onto the bottom wire and turned to see what Lug was up to. I hadn't seen him for some time, and I couldn't remember when I had last heard him wailing over his half-chewed stick. He was nowhere in sight.

"Lug! Here, Lug!"

I wondered where he had gotten to. I was sure he was here when I was digging the last hole. I carried the shovel to the next candidate for replacement. Leaning it upright against the wires, I took off to the clearing in search of my dog. It was unusual for him to leave my side like this. He was rarely more than a stone's throw away.

"Lug! Luuug! Lug, where are you?" My voice had taken on a definite tone of annoyance. I looked toward a cow-calf pair some distance down the gully, wondering if he had decided to torment them with his obnoxious banter. "Lug!" I retraced my steps to the pile of treated posts in the clearing. This was at the top of a little knoll, and I could see for quite a distance in all directions. "Luuuugg! You stupid hound, where have you gotten to?"

I followed the old logging road through the trees toward the Ivany place. I sure hoped that mutt wasn't wandering around bugging John. He was such an orderly sort and not the least bit fond of a change in routine. The last thing I needed was trouble with another neighbour—Verna and I had still not exchanged words since she had chopped off my waterline. I hated the thought of being totally surrounded by enemies.

I crossed the old creek bed and strode up the hill to the spot where I hoped to someday build a house. I stood in the clearing and peered across the road toward the Ivany farmyard.

"Luuug! Luuugg!"

I listened for the telltale ruckus that he made while chewing his stick. Turning in all directions, I strained for at least a hint of him somewhere…nothing.

I marched across the roadway and opened the swinging metal gate that John religiously kept closed. As I walked down the long driveway, I couldn't help but feel somewhat intimidated by the condition of the farmyard. The approach was bordered by a well-kept fence on one side and a proliferative hedge of lilacs on the other. Everything seemed so orderly and manicured. I wondered if my property would ever take on a similar air.

I approached the small white two-storey home that was perched like a dollhouse at the top of a draw. Constructed by John's father, Alex, when they homesteaded the property, it was still occupied by John and his parents. I hesitated for a moment, then knocked on the glass of the aluminum storm door. I heard shuffling inside the house, and within a few moments the inner barrier was swung open by a short, stocky man in his early fifties.

"Good morning, Doctor." He addressed me in his usual formal manner, then smiled and opened the outside door. "How are you this morning?"

"I'm fine, John. You?"

"We're doing better this morning. Mom had a bit of a bad spell yesterday." He ran his hand through his cross-cropped hair.

"Sorry to hear that. Is it anything serious?"

"She gets dizzy spells and took a bit of a tumble. We had her up to Emergency, but they sent her right home." John stood back and held open the door to reveal a clean and orderly kitchen. "Would you like to come in and sit down, Doctor?"

"Maybe some other time, John." I fidgeted uncomfortably at refusing his offer. "I was just hoping that you had seen my dog this morning. I was digging fence-post holes, and the next thing I knew he disappeared."

"Sorry, Doctor, I haven't seen him." His face suddenly became very serious. "I'd go over to Mrs. Levett if I were you. One of her boys was here just yesterday looking for their dog. Apparently she's in season."

I immediately felt weak. I flushed and felt a prickly sensation all up the back of my neck. John smiled a sinister little smile. "I'd be careful, Doctor. You don't want to get into trouble with Mrs. Levett."

"I know, John. I know."

I turned in a daze and took a few steps down the path. "Thank you, John. Sorry to trouble you."

"No problem, Doctor."

I wandered across the yard in a state of shock. At the lilac hedge, I turned to look absently at the house. John remained in the open doorway watching my departure. He was still smiling. I waved timidly, then picked up my pace. By the time I reached the metal gate, my mind was awhirl. What if Verna had shot my buddy? No…I'd been working within earshot of her barn all morning, and if someone had fired a rifle, I'd have heard it.

Consumed with worry, I headed down the main road. By the time I reached Verna's gate, I was about to break into a jog. Forcing myself to slow down, I struggled to regain a bit of composure. If Verna saw me in my present state, she'd be absolutely delighted. I took a deep breath and marched down the long drive to the house. If that woman had hurt Lug, there'd be hell to pay! She could call me what she wanted, do what she would to get under my skin, but she'd better just leave my dog out of it.

I was about to knock on Verna's door when I caught sight of her. Crossing the barnyard with a bucket in each hand, she ducked into the little red building that served as her milk house. Although I was certain that she had seen me, she gave no indication what-soever that she had.

Damn it, anyway. Why did this have to happen? I took a deep breath and headed in her direction. How was I going to handle this woman? I snorted out loud. Was there a man alive who could handle her?

My heart was pounding by the time I reached the squat, win-dowless building. Had she harmed Lug in some way? Did she have him locked up? What if she refused to give him back? I closed my eyes, took several deep breaths, and stepped around the corner. Verna stood with her back to me washing the buckets she had used to haul milk to her weaner pigs.

"Good morning, Verna." My voice was tense. I was sure I detected a tremor and wondered if Verna had picked up on it as well.

"Morning," she responded gruffly. Depressing the trigger on the nozzle of her hose, the woman never looked up. With intense concentration, she continued to pummel the galvanized pails with a constant jet of water. I stared uneasily at the back of her head for several minutes before the water quit. Stooping to dump the metal vessels, she stacked them one inside the other and tossed them with a clatter into the corner.

"I seem to have lost my dog," I blurted uneasily.

"Oh?" Verna glowered at me with burning intensity.

"Have you seen him?" I continued to engage her glare, struggling to maintain eye contact. Her contempt for me was palpable.

"Might have." Verna maneuvered around me in the tight confines of the milk house, then strode purposefully toward the farrowing barn. Again, I felt myself flush. This bloody woman knew where Lug was and was playing games with me. I followed in her wake, getting more and more agitated with each step. I wanted him back...now!

"Verna!" The exasperating woman disappeared into the barn. I floundered after her. My heart was pounding; the back of my neck was burning. What was I going to have to do to get through to this woman? She thrived on this type of controversy, and I was playing her game. Even peering through this veil of pulsating testosterone, I knew that she had me right where she wanted me.

The air in the barn was warm, moist, and heavy with the smell of hogs. I stepped around a wheelbarrow filled with manure and straw and followed Verna down the alley. She stooped to grab a square-mouthed shovel and filled a couple of five-gallon buckets with grain.

"Where's my dog, Verna?"

Resting on the handle of the shovel, she glared at me. "Locked up."

"Why did you lock him up?" I returned the woman's animosity with every ounce of strength that I could muster.

"Caught him screwing my bitch." Verna's features softened ever so slightly, and I detected a hint of a smile. She turned to face me. "Seems we have a bit of a paternity suit here."

I struggled for a response. Verna and I stood only a few feet apart glaring at one another. My mind was whirling. Maybe if I just offered to spay her dog…My eyes wavered and I could see the light of victory flash on in the woman's eyes. She was enjoying every moment of this.

In an instant of total abandon, I took a step toward Verna and put my arm around her shoulder. "Can I please have my dog back, Verna?" She looked at the shovel in her hands as if contemplating giving me a rap with it, then stepped back.

"Take your damn dog and get out of here!" she blurted. "I got work to do and can't be standing around here all day. He's locked up in the calf barn." Grabbing her buckets of grain, she rapidly retreated down the alley.

"Thanks, Verna," I responded almost giddily. "Sorry for the hassle!"

The rollers screeched in complaint as I pulled open the door. Lug bounded from the barn. Dancing around me, he yipped and whined excitedly. He knew he was in trouble but grinned incessantly.

I was so relieved, I couldn't reprimand him. "Okay, you crazy mutt, let's get out of here while the getting is good."

The Other Man

What a relief it was to have a lazy morning. It was after two o'clock and the phone had yet to ring. Lug and I returned from our walk around the block, and I convinced myself that I could just lie back and do nothing. It was hot outside and even hotter in the apartment. There was something about July weather that necessitated a slowdown in activity.

I tore the cellophane from the new Cat Stevens album I had picked up the day before at Sight 'n' Sound and pulled the shiny black record from its envelope. I lifted the plastic cover of my record player, set the record on the turntable, and clicked it to $33\frac{1}{3}$. Adjusting the overstuffed pillow under my chest, I stretched out on the carpet. Life didn't get much better than this.

I wasn't there more than a few seconds when I thought about Sandy. With difficulty, I overcame the urge to go downstairs and check the dog's intravenous drip—I had looked at it ten minutes earlier. What was it that made me feel guilty about even a moment of relaxation?

Cat had only nicely gotten through the lyrics of his first track, "18th Avenue," when the telephone rang. Lug lifted his head from my leg, and I bounded to my feet. I turned down the volume of the recording and answered, "Creston Veterinary Clinic."

"This is Marie Bell," a woman began hesitantly. "My husband and I are travelling from Calgary to Sandpoint on the first day of our holidays…We just got to the border crossing at Kingsgate, and I can't find my dog's rabies certificate. We got it done last November, but I can't prove it now. They tell me here that if you'll

183

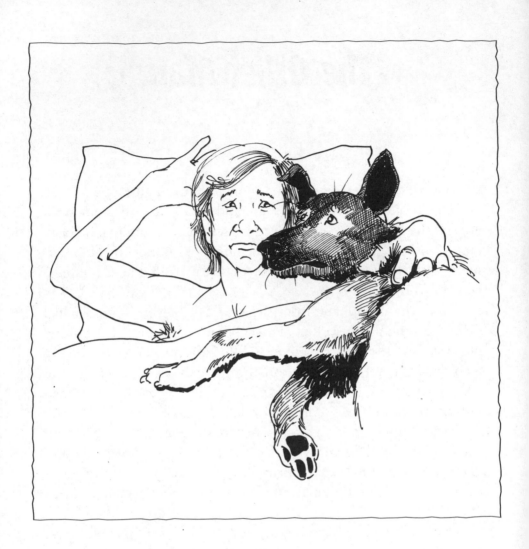

redo the vaccination, they'll let me through." There was an expectant silence as she waited for my response.

"Come on into Creston and I'll take care of it."

"Oh, thank you. I can't tell you how much this means to me,"
the woman blurted. "The last thing my husband asked me before
we went out the door this morning was, 'Do you have Saber's
rabies certificate?' I was sure I knew right where it was."

"I know how that goes. Just come into town. My clinic is
across from the Creston Hotel on Canyon Street—a squat white
building."

I hung up the phone with a mixture of feelings. The part of me
that needed to relax was grudging, but the part of me that didn't
know what to do with my spare time was experiencing a morbid
sense of vindication.

I turned up the volume on the record and once more stretched
out on the floor. Lug dutifully trudged over to me. Collapsing with
his head in my lap, he drew in a deep breath and released it with
a sigh. Why couldn't I learn to relax like him? Why did I take
myself so seriously?

An hour later I was sitting on the waiting room bench staring
out the window. The woman should have been here by now—the
Kingsgate border crossing was only a few miles south of Yahk. As
I fretted, a Lincoln Continental passed by slowly, followed by a
long white trailer. I was jolted to my feet by a sickly crunch and a
horrible scraping sound. Throwing open the door, I dashed out
onto the street. The caravan had come to an abrupt halt halfway
around the corner.

A tall blonde woman in her late forties stepped up on the curb
and ventured around the corner. "Oh God, my husband is going
to have a fit!"

Running her hands through her hair, she paused as if pulling
at her roots. From inside the trailer came a constant racket as a
dog scratched at the door and barked aggressively.

"I told him I couldn't drive this thing!" she wailed, staring up at the white siding that was now streaked with the green paint of the light standard.

I smiled timidly, not certain how to respond.

"What am I going to do now?" she asked no one in particular, still ignoring the complaints of her distraught dog.

"We'll have to get you to cut it hard and back off," I suggested. The barking intensified as I passed in front of the window of the trailer.

The woman I presumed to be Mrs. Bell looked in horror at how the metal pole had gouged into the side of her home away from home. She bit her lip and closed her eyes at the sight.

"You'll have to back it up and swing way wide this time," I said over the increasing din of the barking dog.

"Saber! For heaven's sake…shut up! Things are bad enough without you having a hissy fit."

I ran my hand over the area where the aluminum siding had begun to tear. "Cut it hard the other way and back up," I repeated. "I'm sure you'll be all right."

The woman got uncertainly into the vehicle, and I stood by the passenger door. I twirled my hand around and around until I thought she had the wheels cranked enough, then indicated for her to go back. With a screech of complaint, the metals separated. The woman braked, and I held up my hand while a transport truck loaded with hogs crept cautiously around her.

"Come on back!" I called.

She maneuvered the trailer fifty feet down the street. I motioned for her to swing wide and park on 15th Avenue. As she pulled around the curb several feet from the light pole, I went into the clinic to dig out the book of vaccination certificates and the rabies vaccine.

I waited for five minutes. Still no dog. What was holding things up? I went outside and peeked around the corner. There on the curb, her head in her hands, sat Mrs. Bell. I approached her, wondering what had caused this deterioration of her condition.

"Is there a problem?" I asked hesitantly.

The woman was sobbing so relentlessly that her whole body rocked back and forth. I knelt beside her and rested my hand on her shoulder. "Mrs. Bell, is there something I can do?"

"He's got them," she muttered plaintively. "He's got the bloody keys."

I waited a moment, hoping that the explanation would soak into my thick skull. "I'm afraid I don't understand."

"We were rushing around at home getting ready to leave," she finally blurted between sobs. "We were supposed to be at my brother Bob's in Okotoks by six…We had everything packed and ready to leave Saturday night. The last thing Fred said when we were leaving the house was, 'Do you have the vaccination certificate?'"

She continued to sniffle. "I said it was in my purse…I was sure it was there. When we got to the border, Bob went through first and waited for us."

There was a definite slowing in her tears and her voice raised a few octaves. "I couldn't find it! That's when the Americans sent us back."

She hesitated and looked up at me. I nodded, trying to be taken with the gravity of her situation.

"Fred got so mad at me that he threw me the keys and said, 'See you in Sandpoint!' You see, we had a big fight last night about putting Saber in the kennels. He's my dog really."

I struggled to keep from smiling as she described the scene. I could just picture it all.

"Fred went on with Bob to Sandpoint, and I came back to the Canadian Customs to see what I could do. They gave me your number."

"I can see why you're so upset," I sympathized. "You haven't had a lot of fun yet on this holiday…Just bring him in and we'll have you on your way in a few moments. If you cross here at Rykerts, you'll catch up to them in a few hours."

"But you don't understand!" she shouted. "Fred has the keys to the trailer in his pocket…and Saber is in the trailer."

Suddenly, the reason for Mrs. Bell's hysteria was painfully obvious. I stepped up to the trailer door. The dog barked threateningly. I could see his teeth and toenails slide repeatedly over the window.

I had never really checked out trailer doors before, but this one was poorly designed, with the hinges totally exposed to the outside. I went back to the clinic and returned with a hammer and a screwdriver.

As I tapped away at the pins in the door hinge, Saber tore aggressively at the glass on the other side of the door. "I doubt any burglar would want to get in there when your dog's on duty, but your trailer would be very easy to break into," I told the woman, who was taking deep breaths as if to calm herself down.

Within a few minutes, I had the pins removed and the hinges pried apart at the corner. As Mrs. Bell stood in position to subdue her dog, I swung the door open and let him out. She led the restless German shepherd to the clinic while I lined up the hinges and replaced the door. I checked to make sure it was unlocked, and then slammed it shut.

Saber cooperated nicely for his examination and vaccination. Mrs. Bell loaded him into the trailer and returned to pay her bill. Typical of most bills in the early days of my practice, it was a paltry amount—$12 for the vaccination, $6 for the out-of-hours fee. I handed the invoice to the woman almost apologetically.

Throwing a fifty-dollar bill on the counter, she ran for the door and disappeared to her car. I counted out change from the cash box and chased after her. By the time I arrived outside, her caravan was disappearing down 15th Avenue. A tip! After two years in practice, I had received my first tip.

I poked around downstairs for another hour. After walking Sandy outside for a pee, I changed her blanket and got her settled, making sure that the intravenous was dripping steadily.

Lug and I stretched out again on the floor of the living room, and I was arguing with myself about whether to finish listening to the Cat Stevens record or turn on the television. Somehow, both options seemed to require too much effort to be seriously considered. In this heat, just lying there was enough.

Lug's ears perked up a few seconds before I heard the rattle of the door at street level and the sound of footsteps on the outside stairs. My faithful bodyguard growled and trotted to the kitchen. I got there moments before the knock on the door. I pulled Lug back and peered out the window. There with a big smile stood Cory.

"Hello, stranger," I said, still holding the dog back. "Glad to see you."

Cory smiled and dropped a suitcase at the door. "Do you think you can put us up for a few days?"

"Sure thing. Come on in."

The door below rattled again, and Lug's attention focused on the stairwell. My heart rate quickened and a rush of excitement swept over my body as I recognized the lithe, fluid movements of my other guest.

I smiled broadly. "Marcie! What a treat. I sure wasn't expecting you."

Marcie smiled meekly and stopped hesitantly at the landing.

"I meant to tell you, Dave," Cory said awkwardly, "that Marcie and I have a thing going."

My face felt suddenly hot. I stared at my friend with a look of disbelief as blue eyes searched blue eyes.

"A *thing*?" I blurted.

"Yes…we've been going together for some time now. We're planning to be married."

I blinked. No longer able to meet his gaze, I looked away. Still holding Lug's choke chain, I knelt beside him and roughed the hair on his head.

"Oh."

My heart pounded as I ran my fingers over Lug's silky ears. My face was burning, and I knew from experience just how red my own ears would be. I glanced uncomfortably in Marcie's direction. Her eyes closed, she remained in the stairwell shifting from one foot to the other. I struggled to look up at Cory. Neither of us attempted eye contact.

"Have you guys eaten?" I finally managed to ask.

"We had something in Cranbrook," Cory replied.

"Oh…well, make yourself at home." I pointed toward the living room and the spare room adjoining it. "I'm just going downstairs for a bit to check on a patient."

I headed across the kitchen with Lug at my heels. My mind was whirling. I found it difficult to believe what had just happened.

Was this the Cory who had sat for hours in Saskatoon listening to me babble on about the woman I had fallen for? Was this the friend who had struggled with me through those final gruelling months at veterinary college?

I stumbled down the stairs to the landing and stopped. Lug had already charged to the bottom and stood looking back up at me. I settled on the first step.

How could this possibly be happening? Here I had been worrying away about whether or not there was enough to keep two of us busy, and now there was a third. How could Cory even consider doing something like this to me? He knew how I felt about Marcie. Had he secretly hated me all these years, waiting in the weeds for an opportunity to put me in my place?

The anger struck like a tidal wave. Smashed and buffeted by the wall of anguish and the stress of the last few months, I trembled and struggled to draw a breath. *You rotten son of a bitch. I should just tell you to get the hell out—to haul your carcass as far from me as you can get it! Hell, a real man would toss your sorry ass out into the street.*

I sat on the step with my body tensed and my eyes closed.

190

Cory's words ran through my mind over and over again. "Marcie and I have a thing going." A *thing*, indeed! I'd love to shove *that thing* where it would never again see the light of day.

Lug's wet nose pressing into my hand jarred me from my thoughts of woe. I peered down into his soft brown eyes and took his head in my hands. I began stroking him with a vengeance—focusing on him as if he were the only other being in the universe. Tears welled. I wiped them away with the back of my hand and focused on the dog's sympathetic gaze. He always seemed to know when I needed him. Why would anyone want a woman anyway when he could have his best friend? So long as that best friend was a dog, that is…It didn't seem possible to trust another man.

How could I ever trust that miserable so and so again? How could I work side by side with the man who had taken the woman I wanted? *Oh Lord, why have you done this to me?* I continued to torment myself, running Cory's words through my mind over and over again—re-enacting them—making them carry more weight each and every time I repeated them.

I heard voices near the head of the stairs—footsteps passing through the kitchen. I sprang to my feet and scurried down to the clinic. I had plenty of time to get to the kennel room and open the door to Sandy's cage. I was calmly stroking her head when Cory walked in.

"Has it been busy?" he asked nonchalantly.

"Yeah, pretty."

He stood for several minutes, then reached for Sandy's card and read over the record. "Interesting case?"

"Yeah, sort of. She presented with a history of not eating for a few days and vomiting…I could feel an obstruction."

"You never X-rayed her?" he asked in surprise.

"I could feel the ball as plain as day and didn't see the need for it."

Cory grunted as I handed him the plastic bag containing a little red rubber ball like kids use in the game of jacks.

191

"She's doing fine now, and she'll be ready to go home in the morning."

Cory glanced at the other hospitalized patients and their records. I stood mutely, holding Sandy's head and stroking her fitfully. A few moments later, Cory disappeared and I heard the stairs creak as he ascended to the apartment.

I puttered about for two hours, trying to come up with an excuse for not going back upstairs. Had Cory really thought that I would welcome him with open arms? What was the man thinking? He knew I had concerns about the cash flow with one new person in the practice, never mind two. After all, I handled almost everything that came through the door right now, and Doris still cringed every time we had to drag out the chequebook. How would we possibly make it work with three vets?

It was after nine when I ventured back up. I poked my head around the corner into the living room. Cory was reclined in my velvet chair; Marcie lay stretched out on the floor.

"I'm off to bed, you guys...It's been a long day and I'd love to catch up on some sleep."

I shuffled to my room with Lug at my heels. Stripping to my underwear, I lay in bed with only a sheet covering me. Lug remained on the floor with his head on the edge of the bed. The usual ritual was for him to lie on the floor until I was asleep, and then crawl up on the bed where he could use my body as a pillow.

I lay on my back staring at the ceiling. Although I had pulled the curtains, it was still far too light outside to get to sleep. I watched a brown spider inch its way from the corner over my head across the ceiling. Pausing at the light fixture in the centre of the room, it detoured toward the window. I surveyed the room absently looking for the web, wondering where the creature had established its territory.

Cory laughed loudly. I heard the high-pitched voice of a young man, the canned laughter of a mechanical audience. I wondered what show my guests were watching. I imagined that they sat cuddling on my chair; I was sure they had merged the moment I left them.

I glanced at Lug. He remained at my bedside staring up at me with his jaw resting on the side of the bed. I patted the mattress beside me. He hopped up immediately, not waiting for a second invitation. Treading as far as my shoulder, he collapsed in a heap, his muzzle on my cheek. I hugged him close, burying my face in his coat.

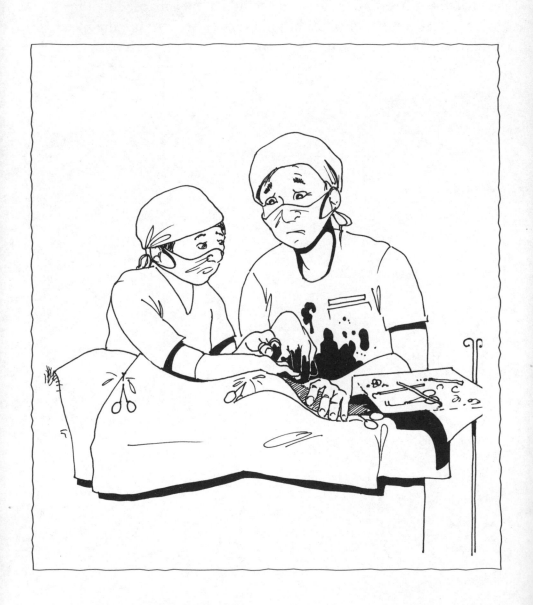

The Final Straw

It hadn't rained at all in the three weeks since Cory and Marcie's arrival, and the daytime temperature hadn't dipped below 26 degrees Celsius. It had been 38 the day before at quitting time, and the intense heat had made sleeping conditions in the upstairs apartment unbearable. Tempers were beginning to flare.

The very sight of Cory fanned the coals of envy until they burned like an inferno in my gut. It was painfully obvious that things couldn't go on the way they were. I couldn't remember a night when I slept more than a few hours. Even wee-hour call-outs became a welcome diversion from the hours of staring at the ceiling and rehashing imaginary conversations with my old friend.

Oh, the battles we had when I should have been lost to slumber—the knock-down, drag-out exchanges. In reality, I had hardly spoken a dozen words with him outside the terse discussion of the occasional case in which our stewardship overlapped.

"You look terrible, Dave." Doris stood solidly in the kennel room door barring my passage. "Why don't you sit down and talk with Cory?"

"Because I don't have a lot to say to the son of a bitch," I responded brusquely.

"Come on, Dave, you obviously have something to say. I've been at your side for the better part of each waking day for the past three years. I know you better than I know my own kids. You're letting this thing with Marcie tear you apart."

I scooped up the little dachshund from the end kennel and tried to squeeze past my tenacious receptionist.

"No, you don't!" Doris snapped. "You're not going to push me aside…You have to deal with this. We can't keep working in this environment. I've watched you endure things in the time we've been together that no man should have to go through. You're one of the most resilient men I've ever known."

"I need to express Princess's bladder, Doris." I pushed my way past her to the sink.

"You *need* to deal with this situation, David." Doris's face had taken on a crimson hue.

I settled Princess on a towel beside the sink, supported her underbelly, and applied gentle pressure to the round structure in the dog's abdomen. Her vulva winked slightly. Urine first dribbled, then flowed freely into the sink. I was sure there was more tone to the dog's bladder today—more resistance to my intervention.

I positioned her hind feet under her and reduced the support from her underbelly. She swayed slightly but remained standing. Not three days ago, the dog had been totally paralyzed from the prolapse of a thoracic disc. Today she looked to be on the road to recovery.

"Princess is looking stronger this morning, Doris. Tell Mrs. Langdon when she comes in that I'm really happy with her progress."

"*Happy*! You haven't been happy about anything since the kids arrived…and don't you dare change the subject. We have to do something about this. I've suggested to Marcie and Cory that they come and stay with me until they can find a place of their own. That poor girl hasn't shown her face around here in days."

"Sounds good to me," I snapped. "I'm tired of listening to their bed springs creaking."

Doris opened her mouth as if to speak. I slipped by her again with the dog in my arms. Grabbing a clean blanket, I folded it several times and settled my patient. Doris studied me, searching for some way of bringing me to heel. She gave up and retreated to the front.

I spent as much time as possible away from the office. Taking every large animal call that came in, I saw none of my associates for the rest of the day. When Lug and I returned, it was to an empty office. I checked the answering machine and clicked it off, looked in on Princess, and was disappointed to find her bladder empty. Cory had obviously expressed it before leaving.

I opened the fridge in the apartment and surveyed all the goodies that Marcie had left behind—the cheese, the sandwich meat, the fresh fruit. I slammed the door with a sense of disdain. Somehow I just wasn't interested in eating—certainly not food that she had bought.

I contemplated my surroundings. Is this what life was meant to be about? Did I want to continue to live in this broken-down dump, waiting to prove to the world that I had something to offer? I should maybe volunteer for CUSO or just go travelling.

I glanced at Lug. The big goof stood looking at me expectantly. His tail wagged rhythmically from side to side—he could care less who bought the food. What would I do with him if I went away? Damn! Life consisted of opening one bag of misery after another.

It was hotter than hell upstairs. I stripped to my undershorts, put on my Cat Stevens record, and crashed on the floor. Maybe now I could relax and really listen to the music—I had yet to hear it from beginning to end. I hadn't sat in this living room for ten seconds since Cory's arrival.

I slipped the headphones over my ears and closed my eyes, listening to the singer belt out the lyrics to "Sitting." "Oh, I'm on my way, I know I am, somewhere not so far from here. All I know is all I feel right now, I feel the power growing in my hair." I wished so much to feel the power in my hair—or elsewhere. Where had my power gone?

The Cat's voice faded. There was a grating sound when the needle lifted from the record, and then only the hum of the turntable. I lay there, not really caring that the record had ended.

Lug was using my arm as a pillow, and his hair tickled as it rose and fell on my skin with each breath he drew. A car engine roared; tires squealed on the street below.

It was hours later when I stirred. I propped myself up and Lug lazily lifted his head to look at me. The telephone was ringing persistently. I rose and stumbled to answer it.

"Hello," I managed groggily. "Dr. Perrin speaking."

"Hello, Dave. This is Steven Halidor. You remember my dog, Brandy? She got hit by a car about ten minutes ago. I wasn't going to bother you tonight—I was sure that she'd be fine till morning, but now I don't know. She ran across the road to meet my son, and my neighbour clipped her...I'm sure from what Frankie said that the wheels didn't go over her, but she isn't looking good right now. I'd sure appreciate it if you'd look at her."

I stifled a yawn. "Was she able to walk immediately after it happened?"

"She hopped to the house on her left leg and looked not so bad to start with. I settled her on her pillow, just to keep an eye on her, you know. I tried looking at her bad leg, but she nipped me. Now she just lies there. It's hard to get any sort of reaction from her. She feels cold...Frankie noticed that first. It kinda scares me."

"Maybe you better load her up and bring her in. It sounds as if she's going into shock. Try to keep from jostling her any more than necessary. I'll be waiting for you at the front door."

Within a few minutes, a new blue Ford half-ton pulled up in front of the clinic. Steven threw open the door the moment the vehicle came to a stop. Swinging his short legs to the pavement, the chunky man rushed around to the back where his son squatted next to a black and white dog. The Border collie lay prone in the box, her head resting on the boy's knee. Although she was covered with dust, and gravel impregnated her coat, the softness of her hair suggested she had been recently bathed. There was no evidence of open wounds.

"You haven't noticed any bleeding?"

Both shook their heads in unison. I rolled back the dog's lip to examine her mucous membranes.

"She's definitely in shock." The pale gums and the slow return of blood to the blanched area beneath my thumb were typical of an animal in circulatory crisis. I ran my fingertips the length of her spine, prodding each vertebra along the way. The dog lay passively, paying little heed to my inspection.

"She only seemed to hurt on the back end?" I asked.

Steven nodded and looked questioningly toward his son. "You said she got hit by the bumper, Frank?"

The pudgy boy nodded passively. "She almost made it all the way across," he insisted. "The bumper just seemed to hit her on the side and push her out of the way. She yelped, though, and sort of fell over when she tried to catch her balance." The boy took a deep breath and paused. His blue eyes focused on his pet as his stubby fingers caressed her muzzle. "I ran over to her, but she took off for the house before I could get there. She hopped on her left leg...The other one just sort of hung there."

I gently lifted the dog's right hind leg.

"Just take your hands from her face for a moment, Frank. I know Brandy really loves you, but sometimes when dogs are in pain they lash out in fear. We don't want to tempt fate."

Frankie leaned back. As he did, his tee-shirt rode up and pale, pendulous rolls of tummy escaped. The boy quickly pulled his shirt down, then brushed absently at the ground-in dirt.

I manipulated the foot, the hock, and the knee without any indication of discomfort. It was only when I shifted the entire leg forward that the dog yelped. Frank jumped. His fair skin flushed; his lip quivered as he struggled to regain his composure.

"It's okay, Brandy," he whispered almost to himself. "It's okay."

I lowered the dog's leg, gently prodded the length of the femur—the thigh bone—with my fingertips. The moment I approached the hip itself, the dog whined and whirled in my direction.

"We'll need to get some X-rays of those hips," I suggested. "I suspect that we have something involving the joint itself—either a fracture or a dislocation."

I pulled a length of cotton gauze from my pocket and slipped a loop over the dog's nose. I tied it on the top and repeated the procedure on the bottom, tightening it and tying behind her ears.

"Just a bit of insurance, girl…I know you're in pain. We'll move you inside where I can get a closer look at you." I dropped the tailgate and gently slid the dog toward me. Gathering her in my arms, I carried her into the office.

In less than half an hour, Brandy was looking much brighter; her colour had returned to normal. The administration of fluids, Demerol, and steroids had produced their usual wonder.

Steven removed the lead X-ray gloves but was still adorned in the apron. The ties—which on Doris encircled the body and tied in front—met nicely in the middle of the man's back. Beads of sweat had formed on his face; his cheeks were flushed. "Can you get me out of this thing?"

"Sure thing…I hope we don't need more X-rays, but if we do we can get you suited up again."

I hung the films on their racks and stared into the darkness. The six minutes it took for developing seemed like an eternity. I hadn't bothered to turn on the safelight for this procedure—I was doing everything by feel. Somehow when I was depressed, darkness had a strange appeal.

It wasn't uncommon for a dislocated leg to produce a grating sound when it was manipulated. There was something ominous about the way this one felt, though. The grating was more menacing, and the way Brandy reacted, I was convinced there was involvement of the pelvis.

I hoped this would be a simple manipulation where the head of the femur plops into place with the first tug and stays without difficulty. I didn't feel up to struggling with a grossly distorted pelvis. How I hated peeling back all those muscles in search of the broken bones beneath. *Please, God, let this be something simple.*

I yawned again—whatever the situation, correction would wait until morning. I was in no shape to be doing anything challenging tonight. Besides, Brandy needed time to stabilize.

The bell rang. I removed the racked X-rays from the developer and dunked them several times in the water bath. Just a few minutes in the fixer, and we'd know for sure. I fumbled with the lid and slid them inside the tank. Sniffing my fingers, I winced at the acrid, metallic smell that would linger for hours. I scrubbed my palms together in the water bath.

I cringed as I held the films up to the view box. Steven and Frank stood on either side of me, staring up at the plastic sheet.

"Oh man," I groaned. "This is not what I wanted to see," I pointed to the rounded blob of material that remained in the hip socket and several other chunks that floated nearby. "This is the head of the femur. It was attached to the rest of the bone, here." I pointed to the long portion that was displaced several inches above it.

"In the dog, the blood supply to this part of the bone comes from the long bone itself, so pinning or screwing it in place almost always fails because of lack of circulation. The best scenario would be to replace it with an artificial joint. The procedure is still experimental, but the results are more and more impressive. There's no question that the best option would be to take her to the veterinary college at Pullman, Washington."

"Is there another alternative?" asked Steven. "That one sounds expensive. We just bought that new truck. Frankie's heading off to summer camp, and things are pretty tight for us."

"There is." I hesitated a moment and thought about the complicated approach to the surgical site through the top of the hip.

"There's a procedure called an excision arthroplasty...It was developed by people doing research into hip replacements. The first few successes were actually experimental failures where the surgeon removed the head of the femur and implanted hardware.

When the implants loosened, rather than destroy the dogs, they just went in and took out the hardware. What they found was that some of these dogs got along famously without further intervention. They even walked without a limp.

"Once the head of the femur is gone, there's no more direct interaction, and the bone literally floats in an artificial pocket that develops in the muscle tissue. Some larger breeds have a change of gait and need more support, but a dog Brandy's size usually gets along very well."

I peered at the lucent blobs of bone, thinking how simple it must appear to the Halidors to just reach in and pluck them out. The thought that muscle after muscle would have to be severed in order to get the most tenuous glimpse of the situation left me exhausted. I recalled a recent struggle to get even the faintest glimpse of the bone at the bottom of a deep well of oozing flesh.

I stared wearily at my text, *Canine Orthopedics*. I had tossed and turned all night worrying about the procedure. How I prayed that Steven would change his mind and arrive first thing with the news that he had decided to take Brandy to Pullman. At times like this, it bothered me that people thought I was so competent—if they knew what was going on inside my mind, I'd probably not have a client left.

I flipped the page back and forth trying to make sense of the jargon. I had read the description a third time before I threw it aside and went to the kitchen. Breakfast was something I could handle today. Frying bacon until it was crisp was easy enough. Breaking eggs into a pan was manageable. Hell, it wouldn't matter whether my egg hit the plate with its yolk intact or whether it was broken and oozing. It would all end up in the same place by the end of the day.

I had checked Brandy several times during the night. It wasn't any great effort on my part—it was a break in the monotony of watching patterns of lights from passing cars as they displaced the shadows on my ceiling.

It was almost seven o'clock when I returned to the living room and glared at the still open copy of *Canine Orthopedics*. I tried to focus my attention on the dissertation—to really glean something from what I was reading. My eyes burned as I plowed on...there were five different approaches to the joint, all having major disadvantages and some small benefits depending on the location of the fracture. One meant chopping off the top of the femur and later reattaching it; almost all the procedures involved the severance of many, many muscles.

The last time I had performed this surgery, I had used the dorsal approach. It just didn't make sense to me to cut through muscles, sew them back together, and hope that they could support the weight of the dog's body. Whittick, the author of *Canine Orthopedics*, noted that he usually used the ventral approach. It made sense to go in through the bottom. That way, the only muscle I had to cut was the pectineus—the firm band I could feel in the groin when I tipped the leg to the side. After separating the muscles under it—the iliopsoas and adductor—I'd be right there at the head of the femur.

Was today the day for plowing new ground? I was feeling nervous as I positioned the dog and clipped the area in preparation for surgery.

"Do you feel this muscle right here, Doris?" I showed her the tight band that popped up the moment I extended the leg. "It's the pectineus. I have to cut through the middle of that and then separate the muscles to get to the hip joint."

"I always thought that the hip was up here." Doris patted her butt.

"It is...but you can also get at it from the underside."

"Humph." She squirted some Bridine on the dog's underbelly and started scrubbing. "You keep coming up with something new."

She worked in silence for a moment. "I got a call from Sonja Wittmoser. Apparently she's expecting you to stop down and look at her new dog."

"Oh yeah, I did tell her I'd be visiting Mom and Dad this weekend."

As I adjusted the ties for my cap and mask, I wondered why I was constantly getting myself into new commitments? Last week Sonja had asked if I'd check over a dog they were considering buying. He was a German shepherd—a Canadian field trial champion. Yesterday she called again. The dog had been delivered but was limping badly on a hind leg. She wanted me to give her and Siggy a pronouncement as to whether or not to keep the dog. The breeder was willing to give them a heck of a deal now, but they weren't interested unless I said he was likely to recover.

Aggressively attacking the dirt beneath my nails with a brush, I wished it was as easy to access and wash away the foreign material from my mind. Brandy was my patient now, and she deserved to be the focus of my undivided attention.

Cory and Shirley were busy with office appointments on the other side of the wall, and I tried unsuccessfully to drown out the man's voice. By the time I had finished my scrub, I found myself straining to listen to the advice he was giving a new client on the care of her puppy. I was annoyed when he moved the woman into the exam room at the back where I could no longer critique every word he was saying.

"How are you doing, Doris?"

"If you're happy with what I've scrubbed, then I'm ready for you. I've gone from here to here." She indicated an area bordered by both knees as far forward as the mid-abdomen.

"That looks good…Paint it up."

Dipping some cotton into an antiseptic solution, she coated the entire area with the reddish-brown liquid. I ran my gloved finger back and forth over the area for the planned incision. Pushing deeply into the inguinal area, I convinced myself that I could feel where the socket would be—the location of the errant chunk of bone that had now become a liability to Brandy's body.

I closed my eyes and conjured up the image of this dog running across a field, stretched out in full stride, her long feathered hair whipping in the breeze. The image faded before she had gone half a step. I felt weary—so unprepared for this surgery. *Please, Lord, guide my hands...Let this procedure be a success.* Conscious of the regular thump, thump, thump of the femoral artery that coursed beneath my touch, I rested my hand there for several moments.

"Are you all right, Dave?" My eyes popped open and slowly focused on Doris. With her cap and mask in place, all I could see was her caring eyes behind the horn-rimmed glasses, but I could feel the intensity of her stare.

"I'll be fine. It's just the uncertainty of another leap into virgin territory."

"Did you sleep last night? It doesn't look like it."

"Not a lot," I admitted. "Found it a bit hot."

I gazed down at the little green book that had gotten me through so many previous journeys into unknown terrain. *An Atlas of Surgical Approaches to the Bones of the Dog and Cat* lay open at page 99. The text recommended an incision in the form of a T, with one extension running in the fold of the groin and crossing the origin of the pectineus muscle.

"Scalpel blade, Doris."

She diverted her attention from my face and fumbled in the pocket of her smock. Producing an aluminum foil package, she separated compressed halves to reveal the gleaming metal within. I grasped the blade and installed it on the scalpel handle. With one smooth stroke, I laid open the skin exactly as the book portrayed, ending several inches short of the dog's vulva.

The second incision was to follow the pectineus and run one-quarter to one-third the length of the femur. I palpated the firm band that represented the muscle and made my incision. Using the blunt end of my scissors, I peeled back the fascia and exposed the underlying anatomy.

Driving my finger deep between the pectineus and adductor muscles, I separated the two bundles and repeated the procedure on the other side. I carefully isolated the band of muscle from the femoral artery, vein, and nerve that ran the full length of the incision. I slipped a pair of curved forceps under the belly of the pecitineus, and with the scalpel severed it through the centre.

"Doris, can you please turn the page."

I opened and closed my hand several times. My fingers were shaking uncontrollably. I couldn't ever remember this happening at the beginning of a surgery. Only at the point of sheer exhaustion had my fingers done this before—or after three or four cups of coffee. Doris glanced worriedly in my direction. I quickly lowered my hands and rested them flat on the dog's leg.

I pushed deeply with my finger into the depression that I presumed to be my destination. I read the description on page 100, then glanced at the diagram on page 101. I pushed further on the severed muscle belly. The mass under my finger had to be the iliospoas muscle; I could now see the long ribbons of the deep femoral artery and vein. I picked at the vessels and elevated them.

My forehead was warm and prickly. I could feel the telltale tickling of sweat running on my face. I leaned back for fear of contaminating my surgery site.

"Doris…could you grab a towel and dry me down?"

I looked back and forth from the book to the surgery site, trying to decide where to resume my dissection. I took a deep breath and read the book again. "The iliospoas muscle lies oblique to the femoral shaft and runs in a craniolateral direction under the femoral and deep femoral vessels."

I prodded at a barely distinguishable line that began under the artery and vein and blended with the surrounding tissue.

I read on. "An interval between the iliospoas muscle and the adductor muscles is developed by blunt dissection." I gingerly opened my forceps, tearing the fascia between the two muscles. Convinced that I was on the right track, I pushed deeply into the hole I had created. I was sure I could define the perimeter of the hip joint.

I had another look at the text before I jammed my index fingers into the hole, hooked them, and pulled them apart. The muscle tore free and I elevated it as much as I could. I swabbed at some blood in the newly created cavern and tried to make sense of what I saw. Was this the rim of the socket—the acetabulum? Was that the end of the fractured bone? Everything was the same colour—blood-red. I felt the smooth edge of the hip socket, then the rough surface of the object within. That had to be the surface of the fracture, and inside was the head of the femur. I ran my finger as far as I could along the margin of the bone and pulled down on the dog's leg with my other hand. Oh man, there was the jagged edge of the other end of the fracture way up there. How in the name of God was I supposed to work on that?

I suddenly felt a flush all over. What had I gotten myself into? My eyes drifted to the last line in the guide under comments: "Exposure of the joint by this approach is quite limited and its use is therefore quite limited." I had read that last night but had chosen to ignore it...Now I wondered why.

"Doris, can you wipe my face?"

I stepped back and Doris reached in with a towel and dabbed at the beads of sweat on my brow.

"Is it that bad?" she asked.

"It's that bad."

I struggled to pull the iliopsoas muscle back out of the way enough to be able to see something. If Whittick could do most of his excisions this way, I could manage this one. I remembered that he had gone on and on in his text about the importance of proper removal of the femoral neck...First things first.

"I need the other textbook I was reading, Doris. It's on

the counter in the lab, the blue one—*Canine Orthopedics*."

Doris checked the dog's colour, had a look at the gauges on the anesthetic machine, and ducked out of the room. Within a moment she returned with the book still open to the page I'd been reading. Using a Kleenex box as a prop, she set the book up on the end of the table.

I skimmed over the diagrams and began reading. "An osteotome, chisel, bone cutters, or Gigli saw may be employed to perform the excision of the neck and head. The instrument used is not as important as the angle at which the head and neck are removed from the shaft of the femur."

How in hell was I supposed to get any of that hardware up in there when there was barely room for the tip of my finger?

I worked my index finger along the margin of the femur and pulled down on the leg. The jagged edge of the neck hooked the surface of my glove. I rotated the leg back and forth, trying to position the sharp protuberance right into the centre of the cavity...If I could just get an instrument up there, maybe I could whack it off flush with the bone.

My eyes wandered over the alternatives in my arsenal. I had had Doris autoclave some wire on the off chance that it could be useful...What a joke to even think of using it now. How could I ever position the wire for the cut needed when I had so little access?

I was left with either the osteotome, which was a glorified chisel, or the bone cutters. I chose the osteotome. It was the narrowest weapon and undoubtedly the easiest to get into such a restricted area. I rolled it over and over in my palm, then put it down...There was something about whacking away with a chisel where visibility was nonexistent that didn't sit well with me.

It would have to be the bone cutters. I opened and closed the implement a few times. The jaws definitely opened wide enough to engulf the neck of the bone, and if I pushed them in closed, I might just be able to position them.

Damn, it looked so easy in Whittick. In his diagram, the entire bone was still intact, and all he had to do was slip the cutters over the neck and snip the head off flush. I elevated the iliopsoas muscle with the fingers of my right hand and pulled with all the strength I could muster on the end of the draped leg with my left. There it was. I could just make out the jagged edge of the fractured neck. Situating the flat face of my instrument right next to the bone, I worked it up as far as I could. Opening the cutters, I pulled down on the leg and positioned the instrument. My hands were cramping and my arms trembling with exertion when I finally squeezed the handles closed. The bone crunched.

I hesitantly extended my forefinger into the cavern. A piece of bone floated freely. I grasped it with forceps and ripped it away from a bit of muscle that still remained attached to its upper margin. Not bad—still a bit rough, but it would do.

"Doris, can you flip the page?"

The text suggested using a small bone rasp to remove any bits remaining on the shaft. If not properly planed, the patient would have pain shortly after surgery.

For half an hour I fiddled and fussed with first the bone cutters and then the osteotome. By the time I had finished, I was satisfied that the surface had been worn as smooth as possible. I displaced the iliospoas muscle as far as I was able to and focused on my next step. The head of the femur was broken flush to the level of the hip joint, and the joint capsule around it seemed to be still intact.

If I could only see the bloody thing…Why in hell did things always have to be so difficult?

I pried the resistant mass of muscle over. My fingers ached and trembled as I worked to maintain even the most precarious view of the socket. I grabbed some forceps and poked firmly against the nearest corner of the hard surface. It definitely moved. My fingers slipped and the muscle reclaimed its rightful position.

"Damn it, anyway!" I was struck by an overwhelming wave of

frustration. I didn't want to be here. I was tired of being thrown into situations where I was expected to deliver the impossible. What difference did it make if I removed this hunk of bone, anyway? I had already done the most important thing. The neck of the femur was smooth and wouldn't cause the dog pain. This bloody little piece of bone was just a floatie. The worst that could happen would be its erosion from lack of blood supply.

I clasped my hands together at my breast and clamped my eyes tightly, struggling to contain the tears. I took a deep breath and held it until I was ready to explode. I felt a trickling sensation on my right cheek. Why did I have to be such a baby about everything? I wanted to be able to wipe the tears away—to hide my shame. I stood there trembling.

Doris's eyes were on me. "Dave…would you like me to give Cory a call? It doesn't hurt to admit that you need his help."

I shook my head.

"Do you remember when we were pinning the leg on that St. Bernard from Crawford Bay?" Her voice was even and steady. "You were having trouble lining it up, and you told me that you couldn't wait until Cory got here so you could have another pair of hands."

She stopped for a full minute. "Cory's here now. He has a good pair of hands…Give him a chance to make this work."

I opened my eyes to consult Whittick. I tried to read on, but the image of the hip X-ray after surgery was all I could see—the socket empty, with no place for bone to rub on bone. I knew I had to remove the floating chunk. Even if it made no difference, I had to remove it. I couldn't leave behind radiographic evidence of my incompetence.

I focused on *Canine Orthopedics*. "The iliospoas must be retracted cranially and the adductor muscle caudally to appreciate the joint capsule. The latter structure is incised, synovial fluid should escape from the joint and the head of the femur will be revealed."

That was all well and good for Whittick. He was talking about an intact bone that he could lever and clip around. With Brandy, everything was flush—like an inserted screw with a broken head. There was nothing to grab onto. Somehow I had to tap it and weaken its connection to the rest of the body.

Separating the muscles sufficiently to see just a crack, I grabbed a towel clamp and drove its sharp, steel tips into the bone. I lifted gently, hoping it would pop free. It didn't budge. Rotating the clamp in circles, I could see that the joint capsule was still mostly intact. I jammed the tip of my scissors under the rim and began snipping away. My fingers slipped; the muscles reclaimed their territory.

"Son of a bitch!" I hollered. Doris looked uneasily toward the flimsy panel door separating us from Cory and his afternoon appointments. She said nothing—the look of disquiet on her face was chastisement enough.

I stopped and stared out the window. Someday this whole procedure would be nothing but a bad memory. Muscles had resisted me before. Muscles would resist me again. I engaged Doris's eyes for several moments. We carried on a mental conversation.

I followed the clamp to its roots, got the best exposure I could, and began snip, snip, snipping my way around the joint. I consulted *Canine Orthopedics* again. Whittick continued: "The teres ligament is now severed…The joint capsule is completely severed in a circular fashion around the neck. The femoral head may now be luxated medially and the neck freed of capsular attachment using a periosteal elevator."

Oh yeah…fine for him to say that when *his* bone was still intact. This would be duck soup, too, if I had the rest of the femur to use as a lever! I poked the point of my scissors deep beneath the head and prayed that it would sever the ligament. When I pried up and down, the joint seemed looser, the bone more mobile.

Whittick mentioned a periosteal elevator. Was he literally prying it out? Why couldn't I do the same? I reached for the osteotome. Why not just pry the sucker loose? It didn't matter if the errant bone came out in one piece or ten, so long as at the end of the day it was gone. I contemplated using the chisel to just whack this thing in half and then remove the pieces one at a time.

I wanted to get this over with so I could head down to Riondel. How great it would be to just relax on the beach. The cool, crisp mountain air of Kootenay Lake would be a welcome change from the sweltering heat of my apartment. I pictured myself running down the beach straight for the water. Two or three giant strides, and I would just throw myself in—bury myself beneath a cool, refreshing liquid blanket.

I squeezed the tool into the socket. "There we go," I muttered as the blade slid into the cavern. I pried up on the handle, hoping that the bone would just pop up and declare itself free. I twisted the blade and struggled against the resistance of the teres ligament…

"Oh shit!"

The ligament suddenly gave way, and the osteotome took off as if possessed. It sliced through my glove and zipped past my finger. Within seconds the entire surgical field was covered with blood.

"Oh no." Instinctively, I dove for the source of the bleeding.

"What happened?" Doris's eyes were the size of platters. She automatically checked the gauges and pressed on Brandy's gums.

"The osteotome slipped. I must have severed the femoral artery."

My hands were shaking convulsively as I struggled to apply pressure.

"Open me some Dexon!"

Doris hastily dug through her smock pocket. "What do you want me to do with it?"

I grabbed the package of suture material with my left hand. My fingers were shaking so badly that it was all I could do to hold on to it. I released the artery for a fraction of a second so I'd have two hands to open the packet. A jet of blood shot across my face and down the front of my gown. I grabbed a gauze and clenched the vessel with both hands.

"Call Cory!"

Doris scurried off and I could hear muffled voices in the exam room. In less than a minute she returned with Cory on her heels.

"What happened?" he took one look at me, grabbed a pair of gloves, and rushed to the opposite side of the table. "How in hell did you cut it way up there?"

"Osteotome slipped."

He picked the package of Dexon from the pool of blood in Brandy's groin and opened it. Grabbing a pair of drivers from the instrument tray, he clamped onto the needle. He pushed his fingers under mine and bent down to inspect the bloody mess. I shut my eyes tightly and pulled my hands away from the site. I struggled for control. *Oh Lord, please give me strength.*

"Damn!" Blood gushed again as Cory made a feeble attempt to drive a suture. "For Pete's sake, Dave...don't just stand there!"

He dammed the flow as I fumbled through the instruments on the tray in search of a hemostat to arrest the blood flow. I grabbed at one with hands that still refused to function. I scooped it up and dropped it on the drape next to Cory's hand. Grabbing a few more sponges, I displaced his hold on the artery.

"See if you can clamp it...I've had it for today."

Working the instrument into place beneath my fingers, he compressed the handles while I numbly surveyed the carnage. I carefully lessened the tension on the blood-soaked gauze and lifted my fingers. The flow seemed to have stopped. The vessel was clamped.

How in hell could I have been so careless? What an incompetent son of a bitch I turned out to be. And what now? We couldn't just clamp off the femoral artery, could we? I wiped away some of the blood and reached for more gauze, but my hands were still vibrating. Cory grabbed it unceremoniously from my hand and daubed at the wound site.

"Don't know how you managed to miss the femoral vein," he muttered.

"We have to do what we can to try and suture that artery," I mumbled in return.

Cory looked at me critically. "You've damn near cut it right off—"

I avoided his gaze. "Please try."

He busied himself with the task. Doris's eyes met mine for a fraction of a second, then flashed back to the surgery site.

"What do you think?" I asked. "Can you fold some of the surrounding tissue over top just to make sure it doesn't leak?"

Cory finished suturing and cut the material. He took a bite half a centimetre from the wound, tied it, and began pulling tissue over it as a supportive patch. He released the hemostat. I was relieved not to see a gush of blood. It appeared to be holding.

"God knows whether I've left enough of a channel to do any good." He shrugged his shoulders, and we both stood staring at the blood-soaked field.

"Can a dog do without the femoral artery?" Doris whispered.

Both of us shrugged. I had absolutely no idea.

"Are you finished?" Cory asked.

"Close to…I was having trouble freeing the femoral head, but if you'll just give me some traction, I can maybe get it done."

I returned to my original battle site and parted the muscles. I indicated the handles of the skin clamp.

"Just see if you can free that up now."

Grabbing the clamp, he lifted the bone fragment. Although still attached at its upper margin, the ligament had obviously released its hold. Cory snipped around the edge to sever the remnants of the joint capsule. In less than a minute, the offending structure was in the garbage can and no more than a bad memory.

"You should be all right now." Pulling off his gloves, he turned on his heel and left the room.

I looked at Doris and shook my head. Reluctantly taking up

the needle drivers, I began closing the wound. By the time I placed the last of the skin sutures I was exhausted…and defeated.

"You can cut the anesthetic, Doris."

She adjusted the knobs on the machine and flushed the bag with pure oxygen. Removing her mask, she regarded me with concern.

"What are you going to do, Dave? I've never seen you like this."

"It's over, Doris…This was the last hurrah."

"Don't be silly. You're just having a bad day."

"You call this a bad day…Brandy'll be lucky if she doesn't lose her leg. I'd call that more than a bad day."

"Quit talking foolishness…you know how much your clients count on having you here. Do you know how hard I have to talk to get any of them to even consider seeing someone else?"

I shook my head resolutely. "Not this time, Doris. When I'm not around, they'll be happy to see whoever's here. Give 'em a few more years and most won't even remember my name…I'll just be the tall vet who was here for a few years."

Doris grunted with disgust and busied herself cleaning up the surgery table. I pulled off my gloves and threw them on the tray. Holding Brandy's right foot, I tried to convince myself that it was the same temperature as the other. What if her leg turned gangrenous from lack of circulation? I'd have to amputate it.

I went to the surgery table and rifled through the drawer. Grabbing a nail trimmer, I cut the toenails on Brandy's bad foot to the proper length, then poised the blade over a part of her nail that I knew would be well into the quick. I stood there trying to convince myself that it was time to find out.

Finally, I depressed the handle. The tip of the nail dropped to the table. I held my breath. Within a few seconds it was followed by a drop of blood and then another. I breathed a sigh of relief and squeezed Brandy's toe to stop the flow. I applied a cautery stick to the end of her nail until the bleeding stopped.

I waited with Brandy until the Saturday morning client traffic died down on the other side of the building. Margaret and Doris finished cleaning up, then left together. Poor Doris would have a lot to fill her partner in on over lunch—their boss was going to hell in a handbasket.

Brandy had recovered to the point of standing. She was out of immediate danger, and as far as I could tell was not leaking blood into the surrounding tissue. She balanced precariously on her good leg. Her right one dangled limply with her toes curled under. How I hoped she recovered completely.

"How is she?" Cory's voice came from behind me.

"God knows…I clipped a nail into the quick and it bled." I didn't turn to face him. "If she recovers, it'll be no thanks to me."

There was a long, uncomfortable silence. I remained seated by the surgery kennel watching my unsteady patient.

"You know it can't go on like this," I finally blurted. "I'm sorry, but I just can't seem to deal with this situation."

"You knew it was over for you and Marcie. You told me that when you were in Saskatoon. Why should it be such a big deal for you now?"

"Maybe it shouldn't be, Cory. You're right…Marcie told me it wouldn't work…but that doesn't make it any easier to take."

Brandy took a halting step forward, then collapsed in a heap. The kennel door rattled as she stumbled into it. She released a long, plaintive moan. "There's a girl." I lifted her onto her other side and settled her on a folded blanket with her wounded limb uppermost. The room was quiet once more.

"What do you suggest?" Cory finally asked.

"This practice has a lot of potential," I stammered, struggling to look Cory in the eyes. "I thought about it a lot before I asked Marcie to begin with. I think a husband and wife team could do really well here."

I paused and continued to focus on my friend's eyes. He looked away and took a step toward the door.

216

"I'll sell you the practice for what I paid for the equipment and the cost of the drugs on the shelf." My voice cracked. "I'm finished here."

I stood for a moment looking at Cory's back. His image blurred. I stumbled around the corner into the lab where I couldn't be seen, struggling to keep my voice as steady as possible.

"I'm going to Mom and Dad's for a bit. Then I'll come back and finish up the arrangements."

"Dave..." Cory began.

I walked through the lab and closed the door behind me. Completely numb, I trudged up to my apartment. Stopping at the landing, I collapsed on the stairs. What had I done? Would Brandy ever use her leg again? Why hadn't I insisted that they take her to Pullman?

I glared at the clapboard walls, at the bare light bulb over my head. The braided wire that suspended it was beginning to fray. Was nothing in this world made to last? I heard the patter of Lug's feet in the apartment. He sniffed beneath the upper door, and I turned to see if I could detect his shadow. He whined and rattled the door with his nose.

Not now, boy...just leave me to my misery. Let me sit here soaking in my failure.

He whined again and scratched tentatively at the door.

"Enough!" I bellowed

I closed my eyes and sat in the silence.

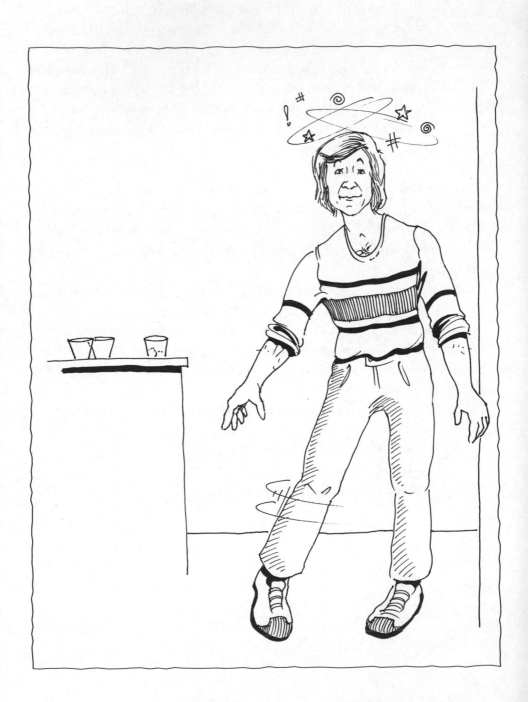

Uncle Doctor and Ike

I was in Crawford Bay making the turn onto Wadds Road before I realized it. Where had the last hour gone? All the way down the lake road, I had been somewhere in the past. One moment, I was in the surgery with blood spurting from Brandy's groin like water from a courtyard fountain, the next I was seeing Cory and Marcie entwined in each other's arms on the living room carpet.

Why hadn't I just jumped into the car and headed for places unknown? As much as I liked the Wittmosers, I was dreading seeing them when I was feeling like this. They were successful business people brimming with confidence and exuding the trappings of prosperity. They chose me as their veterinarian at a point in my life when I had confidence that I could handle almost any problem thrown at me. They wanted the ready-to-tackle-anything guy that they thought I was.

What a joke. What right had I to pretend that I was the man to deal with their new dog's injury? Ike was a champion. How was I supposed to restore him to full function when I had no intention of ever picking up a scalpel again?

I dawdled along Wadds Road, driving slower as I approached the turnoff to the Wittmosers. The road meandered past the beautiful Kokanee Springs golf course. Built almost ten years ago, it was reputed to be one of the most beautiful and challenging courses in Canada. But how would I know whether that was truth or the conjecture of a local enthusiast? The last time I had swung a club was on a Prince George pitch and putt. I ended up paying for a nine-iron that broke in half when I thrashed it over my knee.

I turned left onto a dirt road called Cedar Street that meandered onto a hilltop covered with cedar, birch, and fir trees. I had
visited the Wittmosers several times the past summer when their
house was still under construction, and it would be interesting
to see the finished product. Sonja and Siggy were not ones to let
moss grow under their feet when they made up their minds to do
something.

The road soon turned into a single lane with bush tight to
either side. This was the sort of trail that I usually followed to a
dilapidated trailer or a clapboard shack. Who would expect a man-
sion on the hill with sweeping verandahs and walls made of yellow brick? I pulled into the drive and parked in front of the
gatehouse. I had never seen an estate with an outbuilding like this
before. It was the sort of thing one would expect in the Deep South
or on the outskirts of a major metropolitan centre. I approached
the swinging metal gate and pressed the button on the intercom.

"Yes?"

I recognized Sonja's voice. "It's Dave."

"Come on in."

There was a buzzing sound and I pulled the gate open.
Walking down the curved sidewalk toward the house, I was
impressed with how busy the Wittmosers had been since my last
trip. Red geraniums and dozens of roses of various colours
bloomed in beds beside the walk, and the entire backyard was
the emerald green of a well-manicured lawn. Although the
grass looked lush and healthy, I could still make out the pattern
of the turf blocks that contributed to the appearance of a patch-
work quilt.

A deep-throated bark greeted the chimes when I rang the bell.
Over the barking of the dog, I heard Sonja's lyrical voice.

"That's okay, Ike. It's Uncle Doctor...Uncle Doctor is here to
see you."

The huge oak door swung inward. Sonja was there to greet me,
a very impressive German shepherd at her side. Standing firmly a

half step in front of his new mistress, he watched me intently. His tail flat and still, his eyes fixed on my face, he was an imposing statue. A deep grumble originated from the depth of his throat.

"It's okay, Ike. This is Uncle Doctor. He's going to be your friend. He's going to fix your owie."

"Hello, Ike." I extended my hand, palm up.

The dog sniffed it, then went to work on my lower extremities. Giving the toe of my sneakers a quick lick, he opened and closed his mouth in rapid succession.

"He's picking up on Lug."

"That's enough now, Ike. Let Uncle Doctor come in."

The dog limped off and I stepped onto the tiled floor of the entry hall.

Sonja turned and hollered, "Siggy! Dave's here!"

This woman never ceased to amaze me. Even lounging around her home on a Saturday afternoon, she looked like she was ready to host a garden party. Her hair was neatly coiffed and her slacks evenly pleated. Her green silk blouse had probably been recently plucked from an upscale sales rack.

I slipped off my shoes and followed her into the massive two-storey foyer.

"Where would you like to examine our big boy?" she asked.

"If you can grab a lead shank, I'd like to watch him move."

Sonja retraced her steps to the entry. Grabbing a leather lead from a rack by the door, she clipped the leash onto Ike's collar. The dog wagged his tail madly, excited at the prospect of a walk outside.

"There's a boy, Ike. Let's walk for Uncle Doctor. Show him how you're moving."

"What did they tell you about this injury, Sonja? Has it been bothering him for some time?"

"His handler delivered him here last week." She stopped and turned to face me. The dog immediately sat at her heel and looked up at her for instruction. "Ike was hardly touching his foot to the

221

ground when the man let him out of the carry kennel. We were upset when we saw him—no one mentioned he was injured till he got here."

"Did the handler mention what caused the injury?"

"It apparently happened at the last event—something to do with jumping over an obstacle on the course. He thought Ike must have landed wrong." Sonja glanced lovingly down at the dog. "I hope you can do something for him...We're sort of getting attached."

"I can see that. Take him ahead a bit."

I watched as the dog walked away from me. For the first three steps, he hardly put his foot to the ground. By the time he reached the entrance to the living room, he was using it, but with a decided limp.

"Does he warm out of it? Is it worse after he's been lying around?"

Sonja thought for a few seconds, then nodded. "He's definitely worse after he's been lying down...but it never really goes away. Do you think it could be his hips?" Sonja studied the dog's hindquarters with a worried expression. "Everyone we've talked to has told us it's probably his hips. They say that shepherds are notorious for having bad back ends."

"Hi, Dave!" I turned to face the jovial architect. Crossing the foyer in half a dozen steps, he extended his hand. "How are things with you?"

I hesitated a moment before I answered with a subdued, "Getting by."

Siggy gave me a look of concern. He was about to pursue things further when I spoke.

"Let's just get him on his left side with his bad leg up."

Siggy rushed to his wife's side. "Come on, Ike...there we go, boy." Giving the dog a vigorous rub, he rolled him over and continued roughing up his side. "There's a boy...There's a boy."

Sonja dropped to her knees and held Ike's head in her hands.

"Good Ike...good Ike. Uncle Doctor's not going to hurt you. Good Ike."

I knelt at the dog's side and ran my hand down his leg several times. Grabbing his foot, I palpated each toe separately, spreading, poking, prying the bones apart. The dog lay contentedly. I flexed the hock, rotating the foot first one way, then the other. Nothing.

"Can you tell if it's in his hip?" Siggy asked.

"We might need some X-rays for that...but we should be able to narrow it down without them. This isn't typical of what we see with hip dysplasia, however."

I held the tibia top and bottom, flexing it like a piece of wood. There was no evident pain. I ran my hand over the knee, checking for heat or swelling. Grabbing just below the joint and just above, I straightened the leg and pushed forward with one hand while keeping the other rigid. The dog squirmed and struggled to get off his side. Lifting his head, he thrashed about to get free, then brought it down with a whap onto the tiled floor.

"Easy, Ike. Easy, boy." Sonja's eyes were wide as the dog battled to get up.

"Man, that hurt." I released his leg and patted the back of his head. "That's okay, boy. That's okay."

"What's happened? Why's he so sore?" Siggy straightened and gave the agitated dog a look of concern.

"He has a ruptured ligament in his knee. If you can get me a pen and paper, Sonja, I'll explain what's going on."

She passed me a pen and small pad of paper. I drew out a diagram of the femur and tibia. Beside it I drew a stick representation of a dog's hind leg.

"I'm not much of an artist, so you'll have to bear with me. Now...every time he puts weight on his leg and propels himself forward, there's a net transference of weight from the foot, all the way to the pelvis. You can see how there's a change of direction at the knee. The joint is stabilized with ligaments to prevent the bones from flopping back and forth. The lateral collateral ligament goes from here to here…" I pointed to locations on the outside of the tibia and femur.

"And the medial collateral runs from here to here." I drew in a line connecting the tibia and the femur on the other side. "Inside the joint are two ligaments called the anterior and posterior cruciate ligaments." I indicated them with a pair of crossed lines running inside the knee from the femur to the tibia. "The most important one in the dog is the anterior cruciate."

I glanced at Siggy to see if he was following.

"Ike has ruptured that ligament." I gave the dog a pat on the head and levered him back onto his side. "Hold his head again, Sonja."

Ike was worried; he kept trying to turn in my direction as I again grasped the adjoining ends of the femur and the tibia.

"It's okay, Ike. I'll be very gentle this time." I readied myself, and then applied pressure on the bones to slide them apart. "See how much movement there is—how it slops back and forth when I put pressure on it?"

Both of the Wittmosers wagged their heads in unison.

"The same thing happens whenever he takes a step. I've been told that it's really the stretching of the joint capsule that causes the pain…It would make sense, when a delicate structure is forced to do a job that it wasn't designed to do."

"So what does that mean as far as he's concerned?" Sonja asked. "Is there something you can do?"

"It means that he should have surgery. I'd suggest we do X-rays to rule out anything unexpected…and then surgery."

"How successful is it likely to be? We haven't really bought the dog yet…Will he walk without a limp?"

"I've had very good luck with the cruciate surgeries. There's a little bone on the outside of the femur here called the fabella. With the technique I use, I anchor a synthetic suture around it and drill through the bone over here." I indicated a point on the front of the tibia. "I guess you have to decide how much you like the dog…If he's everything you wanted, I'd give it a shot. If he's just ho-hum and you aren't sure whether he's the dog for you, then I'd ship him back to the breeder and let her worry about it."

"The breeder suggested rest for a month." Siggy rubbed Ike's ears and squatted down beside him. "What do you think of that?"

"If the injury was just causing pain and he didn't have so much movement, or if he were a teacup poodle, he might come along. But a dog his size, with this amount of movement in the joint…" I pensively shook my head. "He's very unlikely to recover spontaneously."

"Oh." Siggy looked at Sonja and then back at the dog.

"I guess giving him a month wouldn't really hurt," I went on. "I'd suggest getting the X-rays right away to rule out a bone chip or something else like that. A month would convince you one way or another if he's the right dog for you."

Siggy glanced at his feet, then at his wife. "I have a feeling we'll be doing the surgery."

"How many have you done?" Sonja asked bluntly.

"At least a dozen," I replied.

"Well—do Ike next. Thirteen is my lucky number."

I suddenly felt uncomfortable with discussing Ike's needs. It wouldn't likely be me doing the surgery anyway. It was one thing to help with a diagnosis, another to actually do it. After all, I was now a man without a practice.

"You've sure come a long way with your house," I said.

Sonja rose to her feet and beamed. "Can I show you around? This is Siggy's dream house—the accumulation of all the good ideas he's seen in houses over the years."

"I'd love to have the grand tour."

"This is the club room," she said, passing beneath a pair of huge oak arches. "And this is the bar." She indicated a long oak bar in the shape of a T. "How do you like our view of the lake?" She held a hand toward the wall of glass through which we could see the entire Crawford Bay area—the creek, the golf course, the lake—and led me onto the balcony that surrounded the house.

"Beautiful." I stood numbly viewing the valley below.

I followed my enthusiastic hostess from one room to the next—the kitchen with its quaint little breakfast nook, the dining room, the sitting room. She led me up an oak staircase to the floor above.

"This is Siggy's studio." She pointed into a room that was clad with oak from the oversize desk to all the trimmings. Never in my life had I seen so much oak. "And this is the lady's den. I've finally got a place to show off the French Provincial furniture that I've collected through the years."

I walked out onto the balcony to take in the awesome view of Kootenay Lake. But Sonja was off again, and I hurried to catch up with her.

"This is Siggy's dressing area, and this is mine…This is the master bath and this, of course, is our bedroom."

I walked into a large room that was furnished much like a living room with a substantial four-posted bed thrown in for good measure. Before I could drink it in, Sonja was off like a shot.

"These are the guest suite bedrooms." She indicated several doors as we passed down a hallway. "And this is Siggy's favourite escape."

I stopped short as I entered the next room. This was the make-believe world that every little boy and probably the boy in every man had dreamed of. There wasn't an inch of it that wasn't dedicated to an artificial landscape. Rolling hills were dotted with grazing cattle. Horse-drawn carts moved down narrow country roads. Miniature houses and churches with steeples lined city streets. Sonja flipped a switch and I watched the scene spring to life—my childhood fantasy—the electric train of my wildest dreams.

"This is Siggy's passion—the German Maerklin railway. He's been collecting and building it for years and finally has a place to set it all up."

I watched in fascination as the train chugged along the track, as crossing arms lowered at the engine's approach. Bells rang; red lights flashed; water flowed.

"Can I offer you a drink?"

I was jolted back to the moment. I had been totally lost in my childhood memories. How many years had I asked first Santa, then my parents, for this very thing. Hell...an electric train with a few yards of track would have satisfied my yearning in those days.

"Sure...I'd love one."

She flicked a switch and the room fell into silence. I reluctantly followed her out the door, and we descended to the lower floor on a wrought-iron circular staircase.

"What's your poison? Gin and tonic? Vodka and clam? Rum and Coke? Rye and ginger? Beer? Wine?"

"Gin and tonic would be great, thanks."

Sonja slipped behind the bar, and ice was soon clinking into a tall crystal glass. I slid onto a bar stool and watched her prepare the drink.

"What would you like, Siggy?"

Not waiting for an answer, she poured gin and tonic for the three of us, then reached into the bar fridge for a lime. She cut several slices, squeezed some in each drink, and dropped a piece into my glass.

"There you go, Doctor."

I grabbed it and took a sip. "You have such a beautiful home, Sonja...And Siggy, you did a great job of designing and blending it in. You have some fabulous views."

Siggy slid onto a bar stool next to me and coddled his drink. "It was a lot of fun working with this site. I wanted to make best use of all the views."

"And tell Dave about your Royal Duchess apple tree, Siggy."

Siggy took a sip of his drink. "When we looked at this property, we just loved this old tree and decided to build right next to it. When we started the excavating, I wouldn't let them get too close. I wanted to have it outside our kitchen window. It's such a beautiful tree—always filled with birds of every description."

"With the lay of the land," Sonja interrupted, "he couldn't fit all the house in…so he stole six feet of my kitchen."

Siggy smiled. "I had to redesign everything…I cut the length of the house back six feet to ninety-two feet."

"It certainly isn't noticeable." I finished the last of my gin and fished the lime from the glass with my straw. I sucked the sour morsel, then removed the pulp with my teeth.

"Well, Doctor, that one certainly went down well." Sonja reached for my glass and began building a replacement. "You're looking tired," she added. "Is everything all right?"

I fiddled with the coaster. "I've had better times."

Sonja regarded me knowingly. "Care to talk about it?"

"Well, you met Marcie one time last summer when you stopped through."

"We did. Nice-looking girl. I remember her well…She was helping you and Doris with some sort of surgery. I thought maybe you two had something going." Sonja finished making my drink and cut another slice from her lime.

"So did I."

I took a healthy slug of the drink she handed me before setting it down. Sonja and Siggy looked at one another, and an uncomfortable silence hung over the room.

"I guess she didn't think so."

I began my tale of woe, slowly spilling the sordid details one by one. By the time I finished, I had lost count of how many times Sonja had refilled my glass. The lime had long since run out of slices to offer and had been replaced by another.

"Would you like a refill, David?"

"No, I better not. I have any more and I won't be driving to Mom and Dad's."

"Well, you're welcome to use the guest room here."

"To be honest with you, I'm getting a bit of a tummy ache. I guess I'm not used to drinking so much."

"When did you last eat?" Sonja inquired.

"This morning…I haven't had much of an appetite lately."

"Well, no wonder…Siggy and I had a late lunch just before you got here. Let me throw a few things together."

"Don't go to any trouble, Sonja. I have to get going soon…I can eat at Mom and Dad's."

Sonja reached over her head for a stubby little glass. She poured a green syrup from a small squat bottle. "Try this. It's great for upset stomachs."

"Crème de menthe? I didn't know it was good for anything but hangovers."

"This is not crème de menthe," Sonja replied in a reproving tone. "This is Jaegermeister. It's a very famous German schnapps made from special herbs."

I stuck it in front of my nose, then touched it to my tongue. It was sweet…and potent!

Sonja retired to the kitchen to prepare a snack while Siggy and I remained seated at the bar. We talked about the economy of the Kootenays—about how the area was the last of the undiscovered gems in British Columbia. I was finding my tongue just a little rubbery, my thoughts a bit hard to express.

Siggy was certain that the east shore of Kootenay Lake was in the early stages of a boom. He was so sure of it that he was going to bring materials in from Calgary and establish a builders' supply in Crawford Bay.

By the time Sonja returned with trays of crackers and meats and cheeses, I had finished my German crème de menthe. She refilled it without comment and I dug into the goodies.

"Eat up, Doctor. Try this Greek feta—we get it from a deli in Calgary—and this Bavarian sausage. Have you tasted the crackers?"

I stuffed myself and Sonja refilled my glass so many times that I lost count. I was finding it more and more difficult to follow the conversation—almost impossible to add anything to it. I turned on my stool. It was time for a bathroom run. My foot slipped from the metal railing and I fell hard against the wall. I leaned against it a moment, trying to gather my bearings.

"Are you all right, David?"

I stood stock-still trying to focus on Sonja's face. The room was moving unsteadily in a clockwise direction. I was finding it difficult to respond to her.

"That German crème de menthe's potent stuff," I heard myself mutter.

"Jaegermeister is 45-proof." She gave me a concerned look. "How's your tummy."

Tummy? What tummy? I closed my eyes and held onto the wall.

"I think I should head out to Riondel...My parents'll be wonderin' what'sh happened to me." I fumbled in my pocket for my keys and promptly dropped them on the floor.

"Damn, that stuff'sh potent..." I mumbled.

"Maybe I'd better give you a ride home," Siggy offered.

"I can..." I bent over to pick up my keys but lost my balance. "Man, that German stuff ish potent..."

"I'm Swami Radha"

"Dave! Dave…it's the phone for you." Father's voice cut through a deep, thick fog.

"Tell them to go away," I moaned. "I don't want to talk to anyone." My head was pounding. I belched and shivered convulsively as I revisited the green liqueur that Sonja had poured into me the night before. Lying in bed with my eyes closed, I pulled the covers over my head and tried to focus on something other than the pain. Tug stirred from his spot in the corner to rest his head on top of the covers. It was well past his usual walk time.

"Go away, boy."

All I wanted to do was sleep. The way I felt now, I could sleep the rest of my life away. I heard the uneven shuffle of Father's footsteps in the kitchen. He muttered something unintelligible to my mother. A few seconds later I heard his voice at the door.

"You better take this."

I groaned and threw off the covers. "Who is it?"

"It's Martha. She says it's an emergency."

"Oh no," I groaned. Something must be bungled up with Brian and child welfare again. No wonder our taxes were so bloody high—with all the red tape involved in getting something as simple as this sorted out. Why couldn't they just get on with it?

"Hello, Martha. How are you this morning?" My voice was hoarse; even I could detect the weariness, my lack of enthusiasm.

"I…I've got terrible news, Dave." I shifted the phone uneasily. I had never heard this tone in Martha's voice before. "It's Brian…He was killed last night in a car accident."

231

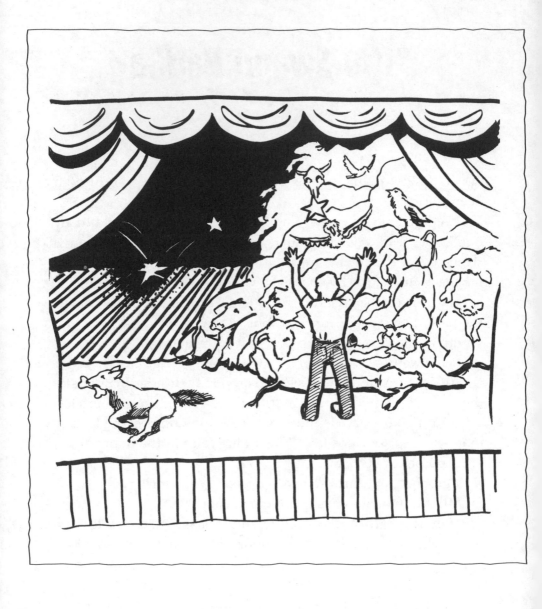

I was dumbfounded, unable to respond. Martha rambled on fitfully. "He arrived on the bus yesterday morning…He insisted that I not tell you when he was coming—he made me promise. The boy was so attached to the idea of surprising you."

A sob exploded from somewhere deep within me. I stood like a zombie as I listened to the poor woman struggle on.

"He walked all the way in to your clinic looking for you. When he found you weren't there, he met up with a couple of buddies from school. He called and asked me if it was all right to go down to Twin Bays…I didn't know that there'd be any drinking, Dave…honest I didn't."

We both wept unabashedly. Finally, Martha said, "Apparently, the boy he went with left to take his girlfriend home. Brian got a ride with a different boy in the back of a pickup truck. They went over an embankment somewhere after Sirdar…I don't have it all straight yet, but for some reason they didn't even find Brian's body until hours later. It sounds like there was a lot of confusion as to how many were there. One other boy died. There's a girl and a couple of boys in the hospital…I don't know how bad they are."

Her voice trailed off again. "I'm so sorry, Dave…I know what John and Brian mean to you. I couldn't feel any worse about it myself."

I was struck by another wave of remorse at the thought of John. How in the world would the boy be able to handle this? Brian was all he had left in the world, and the boys had been so close. To the best of my knowledge, no one had ever found out where their mother had gotten to.

"What about John?" I asked.

"I got hold of him last night…He's on his way here now. He wanted to talk to you right away, but I've had the devil of a time tracking you down. I finally got hold of Doris, and she gave me your dad's number."

Father sat at the kitchen table absently twirling a spoon around and around inside his coffee cup. His eyes were moist as he stared across the room at me. Lug repeatedly nuzzled his nose under Dad's hand, and he rose to take the dog outside.

I closed my eyes, trying desperately to picture the boy who had so infiltrated the fabric of my life—it just wasn't fair that I'd never see him alive again. I struggled until I could almost visualize his face—his winning smile, his big blue eyes, his shaggy blond hair. Just when I almost had him in focus, I burst into tears.

"It's my fault, Martha," I blurted. "You know it is. If I had minded my own business, the boy would still be in Alberta—he'd still be alive."

"Don't talk like that, Dave," Martha protested. "We did the best we could for the boy. Who was to know that something like this would happen? You better get hold of yourself...John'll be back here this afternoon, and he's going to need you. Like it or not, we're all the boy has."

"I'll get back to town as soon as possible, Martha."

Several moments of uncomfortable silence passed as we both searched for something meaningful to say. Finally, I thanked her for contacting me and mechanically hung up the phone. Wandering in a daze, I found myself in the tiny spare room where I had spent the night. I leaned against the bedroom door to close it and pulled down the blind to shut out the morning sun. I looked in disgust at the shafts of light that sneaked in past the curtains. I threw myself on the bed. I wanted to be in the dark, to be alone, to never see light again. I buried my face in the pillow and pounded my fists against the mattress. This couldn't be happening.

"Damn it, Lord," I moaned. "What have I done to deserve this? Haven't you stacked enough on me already?"

Half an hour later the phone rang again. I had reached a point of near numbness, one moment dragging air through the feather pillow, the next convulsing with paroxysms of sobbing.

There was a timid knock on the door. "It's the phone, Dave." My mother was obviously reluctant to bother me.

"Not now, Mom." I felt like a pouting child. Poor Mother—

she and I always seemed to be at odds over something.

"I told him you were not well," she replied hesitantly. "But he insists. He says it's important. It's the new vet you hired."

What was that SOB after now? I slowly lifted my head from the pillow. Hadn't he got everything he wanted already? What did he expect me to do, throw my car in for nothing? I took my time getting to the phone, and when I finally picked it up, stood looking at the piece of plastic as if it were something vile and untouchable. I took a few deep breaths.

"Yeah?"

"There's a call down the lake just a few miles from you—it's a calving."

"So what do you want me to do about it? You're on call. I told you I was finished. It's your practice now…You better get used to working for a living."

"I've got the whole morning booked here. I can't just take off," Cory said impatiently.

"Well, you better make some arrangements with your sweetie then. If you're going to run that place, it's high time you got used to a bit of inconvenience."

There was an uncomfortable silence, and I prepared myself for a blast. I was ready to have it out with him. I had had about all I could take. His response caught me off guard.

"The call is at a place called Yasodhara Ashram. They're having problems with a heifer. Her membranes have been hanging out since five this morning, and she doesn't seem to be making progress. Their number is 227-9224. Call and tell them you can't come. This is still your practice—it's up to you."

I was about to unload a full broadside on Cory when the phone went dead. I listened to the annoying sound of the dial tone and had an overwhelming urge to slam down the receiver. The memory of my wall phone at home dangling from but a few colourful wires flashed through my mind. Not again—not now. I gently replaced the phone on the hook and slumped into a chair by the kitchen table. This drama didn't want to end.

Mother peered out from the living room. "Do you want to talk about it, Dave?"

"Not now, Mom. Sorry, but I just can't handle it at the moment."

I shuffled to my room, sat on the edge of the bed, and held my head in my hands. Crawling under the covers, I pulled them completely over me and closed my eyes. I just wanted to go back to sleep and get away from all of this. Maybe I was in the middle of some sort of nightmare and everything would be different when I woke up again. For five minutes I persisted, tossing this way, turning that. Finally, I gave up on sleep, threw off the blankets, and grabbed my jeans. Like it or not, this day was unfolding and dragging me along with it.

In the bathroom I fumbled through the medications until I found a bottle of Aspirin. I threw four to the back of my mouth, then turned on the cold water tap and stooped to drink. I put the plug in the sink and allowed the bowl to fill. Taking a deep breath, I lowered my face into the water. It had been a long time since I had felt this hungover. I had been in Creston for three years and had only let myself get into this shape a few times. It would be a long while before I'd allow it to happen again.

I came up for air, held a towel under my chin, and headed for the shower. The thought of that heifer was beginning to bother me. If she had been at it for five hours and still hadn't produced anything, there was obviously a problem. How could I sit here feeling sorry for myself and leave her in trouble?

I held my dripping head over the bathtub and adjusted the taps. When the water felt inviting, I stepped in and relished the sensation of warmth over my body. There was something so decadent about this morning ritual. I ducked to bury myself in the flow of water, trying to focus on the warmth, the tingling vibrations against my skin. I turned my face into the flow and concentrated as the water beat against me, tearing open my eyelids and pelting the brow of my nose. I prayed for one moment of silence, one break from this overwhelming pain.

I dried myself and got dressed. I almost hated to admit that I felt somewhat better after my shower. There was a part of me that wanted to cover my body in ashes—to beat it with branches—to really get down and wallow in the absolute depths of despair.

I had to do something about that heifer. There was no way I could just leave the people at the ashram in a predicament. I headed for the door, then stopped. I could call Hugh Croxall, the vet in Nelson, and have him look after it. I put my hand on the phone, then hesitated. This was Saturday—Hughie was probably even busier in Nelson than Cory was in Creston. Even if he could leave right now, he'd have to wait for the next ferry and be hours getting here. I sighed. *Just get on with it—jump in your car, drive over there, and be done with it.*

"Oh no," I moaned. I had been so hammered last night that Siggy had had to drive me home. My car was still at his place.

"Dad! Can you give me a ride to Crawford Bay to get my car?"

The turn to the ashram was on the road to Riondel, just half a mile in from Highway 3A. I slowed as I approached it and turned to the left. I took my time meandering down the dirt drive. A bulldozer had recently rearranged some of the contour of the road, removing several of the switchbacks that I recalled from my last visit. I had been to this place several times and had never gotten much of a handle on what it was all about. I gathered that it was some sort of a Far Eastern–style commune that attracted a lot of hippies.

The road followed the contour of the land through a thick forest of cedar, fir, and larch trees interspersed with occasional clumps of birch. I drove into an opening that had been carved into the hillside and parked the car in front of a squat white building that housed the office and a small bookstore. I had browsed through it the last time I was here to pregnancy-test their Jersey cow. I remembered a bunch of Buddha-like statues and a huge selection of books on Eastern philosophy.

The door pushed inward with a tinkle of a bell. I was immediately met by a good-looking blonde woman in her early twenties. Short straight hair framed a discerning face. She wore no makeup and was devoid of jewellery other than a necklace of brown beads that hung around her throat and disappeared beneath the neckline of her white blouse.

"You must be the vet," she said with a smile. "Ron told me you would have to duck when you came through the door."

I had managed to keep from crying most of the way down the ashram road and hoped that my eyes didn't look too bloodshot. I struggled to muster a bit of a smile in return.

"He's waiting for you down at the barn…Said you'd know where it was. He has water down there already."

I nodded and returned to the car. I drove past a white metal gate that had been left open in anticipation of my arrival. The roadway dipped next to an old orchard, then climbed to a knoll where a group of people were on their hands and knees weeding a respectable-looking garden. A man in his early forties waved as I passed. I raised my right hand from the wheel in response, wondering what he was doing here. I guess hippies came in all ages.

I pulled up next to a clapboard shed in the middle of the garden and recognized Ron. He was a pleasant-looking guy about my age with curly locks that hung down to his shoulders. A slight, white-haired woman stood off to the side of the corral. She was dressed mostly in white with an orange wrap that crossed diagonally on her chest. How in the world did she fit in with all this?

"Pumpkin's been pushing since five this morning," Ron asserted with a look of concern. "I haven't been around many cows when they deliver, but they told me at your office that something should be happening by now."

I nodded to him as I got out of the car. "So there's still nothing showing?"

"Just those membranes hanging down. We had a hard time getting her pregnant. The technician from Nelson came here four different times, so we aren't sure exactly what's going on. It's only been seven months since her last breeding—we weren't expecting her to calve until late July."

I opened the back of the car to remove my gear. Throwing the birthing chains in the bottom of the bucket, I added a healthy slug of Bridine and passed the bucket to Ron. "You can fill that halfway up with warm water, if you will."

I assembled my calving jack as Ron dumped water from one of his buckets into mine. The heifer lay comfortably on her belly near the corner of the corral. In good shape, she appeared typical in size for a Jersey calving for the first time. Although she pushed occasionally against the membranes hanging from her back end, she was still chewing her cud and had a look of complacency about her.

"How old is she?"

"Almost three."

"What was she bred to?"

"Guernsey," he replied. "The technician thought it should make for a fairly easy calving."

I climbed through the rails of the corral and approached the heifer. "Do you think she'll stand?"

"She's been up and down all morning, so I can't see why not."

I patted the heifer firmly on the side. She turned her head in my direction, giving me a detached look. Ron pulled on her halter for a second, then ran to the barn and returned with a bucket of grain.

"I'm afraid she's a bit spoiled," he said with a smile.

"I can see that." The creature stretched her neck in the young man's direction, reluctant to surrender her posture of repose. I lowered my knees to her ribs with a sharp jab. The heifer lumbered to her feet, then twisted her neck in my direction with a gaze of admonition.

239

"Can you tighten her up?"

Ron unfastened the rope that secured her and stood by her head scratching her forelock. I grasped her tail and stretched it as far as possible toward him. "Could you hold her tail for me?"

Ron moved to the animal's side and grasped her furry tassel. I scrubbed the vagina and slipped my arm into a plastic shoulder-length sleeve. The exposed membranes had a pale, half-cooked appearance. Either she had already delivered somewhere and the calf had wandered off, or this calf had been dead for some time inside her. Scratching her tailhead with my left hand to distract her, I slipped my right through her vaginal lips and forward to the edge of the pelvis. My fingers ran into a tiny tail and the pointed brim of the calf's pubis.

"Your breeding date was right. For some reason, the calf is being aborted early."

"I was afraid of that," Ron replied gloomily. "And we have such a problem catching her in heat."

I pushed forward on the calf's butt and slowly manipulated a long, spindly leg from the floor of the uterus.

"The calf is breech with both legs trapped up front—or she would have delivered it on her own."

Ron nodded and glanced toward the white-haired lady who had yet to say a word. I dragged first one hind leg then the other into the light of day. As I applied traction, the fetus, less than two-thirds the size of what one would expect for a term calf, slid easily out. I supported its weight and deposited the body on the other side of the corral wall.

"Have you vaccinated the cattle for I.B.R yet?" On my last visit, we had gone over the procedure for protecting the animals from the virus.

Ron nodded. "I squirted that stuff in their nostrils."

I checked for an additional calf and for any other problems. "Everything else feels fine."

I finished cleaning up my bucket, and Ron and I discussed the possibilities of the cow's abortion. The only other animal in contact with her had calved normally the month before and seemed healthy. Pumpkin's temperature was normal, and she certainly had a great appetite. We decided not to submit the calf to the lab, and I packed away the last of my equipment.

"Would you like to come in for tea?" It was the first time the white-haired woman had spoken. Her voice was soft yet assertive. She had a fairly heavy accent.

"No, thank you," I replied.

I walked around to the driver's door and withdrew the metal container that held my invoices. I quickly scratched out a bill and handed it to Ron.

"Won't you come in for tea?" the woman persisted.

I smiled uncomfortably and declined a second time. I was struggling to suppress tears. I felt as though a heavy black cloud had suddenly engulfed me. I slipped into the driver's seat, smiled half-heartedly at the pair, and slammed the door. Starting the engine, I shifted into first and was about to release my foot from the clutch when there was a metallic tap on the glass. It was the woman again. I was having trouble disguising my agitation as I rolled down the window.

"Are you sure you won't come in for tea?"

I flushed. This woman was beginning to get to me. How many times was I going to have to say no?

"I really have to go," I said brusquely.

A look of incredulity crossed Ron's face. I wasn't sure whether it was because I actually refused the woman's invitation, or because he was astonished at her insistence. I lifted my foot from the clutch and the vehicle slowly moved forward.

"Death isn't the end of everything!" She had raised her voice to be heard over the roar of the engine.

I depressed the clutch and the vehicle came to a stop. "What did you say?" I stared at the woman in disbelief.

"I know that someone very close to you has died. I can feel

your pain." Tears began welling once more and I looked away. "That's the only reason I'm out here," she went on. "If you knew me, you'd realize that I normally don't have anything to do with the cattle. Come in for tea. You have the weight of the world on your shoulders."

I took a deep breath and turned the key in the ignition. With the death of the engine, silence engulfed us. Tears trickled down my face. Peering straight ahead through the windshield, I brushed my sleeve over my face, then clamped my eyelids tightly together in an attempt to seal the flow. My heart was pounding; the muscles of my throat and chest ached in spasm. Why didn't I just leave? Did I want to go into the house of a total stranger and make a fool of myself?

I glanced over my shoulder into the expectant face of the woman. She smiled gently in reassurance, then headed down the roadway with Ron at her elbow. I sighed resignedly and got out of the car. By the time I had removed my coveralls and exchanged my boots for shoes, the two were well ahead of me. I followed briskly down the lane, catching them as they turned toward a sprawling ranch-style house built on the brow of a knoll overlooking the lake.

As I fell into pace with them, I noticed that Ron held the lady's arm as if he were assisting his grandmother. There was a feeling of deep respect and intimacy between them and something special in the young man's eyes—almost reverence. As he opened the door for her, I studied their faces closely, wondering if they truly were related. Entering an alcove, my long-haired friend supported the woman as she sank into a chair. She sighed deeply as if in pain, then straightened herself resolutely. I stood back when a thin, dark-haired woman flitted from the interior of the building and bent to remove the woman's boots.

"Excuse me." I was forced to take a hesitant step to the rear as Ron brushed past me and retreated toward the road. My face grew hot with panic; I focused on his fleeting form. I was possessed with a sudden urge to run. I hadn't expected him to abandon me to these two matrons—at least he was a familiar face. Why was I doing this, anyway?

"Rita, this is Dr. Perrin." There was the slightest tremor to the woman's voice as she shifted in her chair. "Doctor, I'd like you to meet my assistant, Rita."

"Glad to meet you, Rita."

Rita nodded and was about to speak when the older woman went on. "And I'm Swami Radha."

I nodded hesitantly. "Glad to meet you, too." Actually, I was a long way from being glad. I felt trapped.

"Won't you come into the living room? Rita, the doctor's going to stay for tea."

Rita smiled, helped the swami to her feet, and escorted her through the door. "Come, come." The swami smiled reassuringly and gestured for me to follow. I wondered at the woman's accent and guessed it to be German—definitely middle European. With one more hesitant look at the door, I followed after them.

We walked through a cramped hall into a large open room. Everywhere the walls were decorated with Eastern art. Statues of strange-looking idols with multiple heads and arms abounded. I looked around uncomfortably.

"That's Ganesha," the swami said when she saw me staring at a bronze statue of a husky man wearing the head of an elephant. I looked away quickly as if caught snooping through her personal possessions. The last thing I needed was for someone to try and convert me into worshipping some weird elephant icon.

Rita helped the swami into a chair and retreated. I was so uncomfortable. Why had I not just kept on driving?

"Sit down, Doctor, sit down." She waved me to a seat on the sofa across from her. "Rita will have the tea here in a moment."

There was a long silence as I stared resolutely at the white carpet under my feet. When I finally looked up, it was into dark, knowing eyes. Nestled in a high-backed chair that dwarfed her, the woman peered at me as if she were staring into the depths of my soul.

Rita entered the room, set a cup of tea next to the swami and one on the table in front of me, and left without comment. Swami Radha studied me for several minutes without saying a word. I fiddled nervously with the cup and took a sip of the steaming beverage.

"Would you like to talk about what has happened?"

"I just found out that a boy that I adopted as my little brother has been killed in an accident."

At first my words were hesitant. I would mutter a few things, then look back to the tiny woman in the big chair. Before I knew it, I had told her the whole story—the saga of the cows that kept dying one after the other despite my best efforts, the fact that a drug I was selling to my own clients was the source of all their problems. I rattled on about Marcie and how I had felt betrayed when she turned up with Cory. I talked about Brian and John and how it was so unfair for such fantastic kids to be dealt so many bad cards.

Rita made the rounds with a fresh pot of tea. I glanced at my watch and couldn't believe it was after one—I had been talking for over two hours. The whole time, this miraculous woman hardly twitched. Her intense eyes were trained on me as I spilled forth the story of my life. Only occasionally did she speak to ask a question. Never did she comment on my perception of things—never did I feel as if I were being judged.

"Maybe we'll have some lunch. I'm sure the doctor must be getting hungry." I was about to protest when the swami gingerly got up from the chair and made her way from the room.

I sat alone, sipping at my tea, reflecting on the experience that I had just gone through. Never had it felt like anyone had listened more attentively to what I had to say. It was as if this swami had been listening with her whole body and not just her ears. It was as though because I had shared my story with her, she had borne some of my suffering. There was no doubt that the load I now carried felt a lot lighter.

We ate lunch in silence and returned to the living room. Swami Radha was once more seated in her chair. She looked tired. Taking several deep breaths in a row, she sat for a moment with her eyes closed as though regaining her focus.

"From what you've told me, it sounds like you and the boys had some great times together."

I nodded.

"We need to be thankful for special moments," she went on.

"I am, but I often took the joy out of those moments by doing something stupid—by getting angry or by not paying attention. When the boys worked for me, I was a pretty hard taskmaster. I should have given them a lot more credit for what they did well. Now that Brian's gone, I wish that just once in the time that I was with him I had told him that I loved him."

I flushed and my eyes wavered—I couldn't believe the words that had come out of my mouth.

"How often when you were growing up did your parents tell you that they loved you?"

For several minutes, I sat silently returning her gaze. I thought back to those years in our little hamlet of Casino, trying to remember one time that someone—anyone—had told me that they loved me. Tears flowed again as I came to the realization that I couldn't remember a single time.

I looked away and slowly shook my head. Overwhelmed by that old feeling—that deep-down longing—I wanted to get up and run. I stared into space, fighting desperately with the lump that had developed in my throat. How could I possibly explain how I felt? How could anyone, swami or otherwise, possibly understand? It was as if I was missing a special piece—that one piece that would make me loveable.

Swami Radha's voice cut through the fog that had enveloped me. "Most people blunder through their lives as creatures of habit,

David. You were just treating the boy the way you had always been treated."

I stared again at the carpet, somehow unable to handle the continuous intensity of her scrutiny. I had never encountered anyone like her. Looking into this woman's eyes was like looking into a deep, dark pool and knowing that I would not be able to see to the bottom.

"Do you think that your parents love you?"

"Yes. And I know they're proud of what I've done."

"How do you know that?"

"Just the way they treat me. I'm not trying to tell you that my parents have been mean to me or never cared about me. If anything, I guess being the last one at home, I was spoiled…but I don't remember their hugging me. I don't ever remember their telling me they loved me."

"Can you see, David, that your parents were the product of their environment—just as you are the product of yours? You can't blame them for that any more than you can blame yourself. Habits and responses to stimuli are the product of your childhood. It's almost as if your father inherited a pair of crutches from his father as a means of getting around in life. He's passed them to you. If you use them long enough and depend upon them, you'll lose faith in your own legs and constantly have to depend upon the crutches to help support you."

I took a deep breath and wiped my face with my shirtsleeve. Swami Radha passed me a box of Kleenex, but I indicated that I didn't need them.

"If you know that your parents love you, do you think Brian could have known you loved him?"

I looked plaintively in her direction. "I certainly hope he did. He and his brother had such a rough go."

There was another prolonged silence.

"You could make conscious changes in your behaviour, David. You could learn to express your love."

Swami Radha had a look of serenity about her—a look of, for lack of a better word, love. Why did I find it so difficult to engage those eyes? When I looked away, she began again.

"We have to learn to love ourselves before we can truly love another. I came from a home that had many similarities to your own. I know what you speak of."

I leaned back in my chair and stared at the ceiling.

"Did you and Brian ever do anything really fun together? Go anywhere that had a special significance to you?"

I thought immediately of our hike to Meachen Lake, how after several days of following the Goat River and Kianuko Creek, we had finally camped on the shores of a beautiful jewel of a lake nestled below Haystack Mountain. Brian had caught dozens of fish there—I had never seen the boy happier. I nodded my head.

"Picture yourself there now. Go on…close your eyes and picture the boy there with you. Do the things that made you happy then—that made him happy."

I leaned back in the chair, closed my eyes, and we were there. I watched us set up the tent. I watched as Brian and I gathered old man's beard lichen and tiny dry sprigs from the surrounding trees. I saw him get a roaring fire going—he was so proud of himself. I pictured him picking out the lure he wanted to use and me showing him how to tie a fisherman's knot. I watched as a cutthroat trout rose from the lake bottom to grab his hook. I felt his joy—felt mine—all over again.

"Can you still see the boy?" Swami Radha prompted hopefully. I nodded. "Then tell him you love him."

The image faded immediately. I hastily opened my eyes and looked into the swami's gentle gaze. Her intense brown eyes, her delicate features, her white hair slowly blurred. Tears again threatened. I shook my head in dejection and focused on the white carpet.

"Did you come from a religious family, David?"

I shook my head. "I was confirmed an Anglican but never

really had much to do with the church. I went up for communion three or four times, then abandoned it."

"Do you feel as if you have a connection with the Divine?" she asked.

"No, I guess I'm sort of an agnostic. I don't spend a lot of time thinking about God. Sometimes when I'm alone with nature, I get the feeling that there has to be something in control of it all. When I'm at an isolated lake and there's not another living soul around for miles and miles, I feel a bond with something."

"You work with animals all the time. Don't you feel a life force that runs through them? Aren't you amazed that all those body parts and organs are made up of millions of cells working together in perfect harmony? How could that happen by accident?"

I shot a timid glance in her direction. "I can't help but wonder at times…especially when I'm around at the time of death. There's something that happens when an animal dies. It's the eyes—that indefinable light that fades. When you put a critter to sleep, one second it's there, and the next it's gone."

"So what do you think happens to that light, David?"

I shrugged. How could anyone know what happens to it?

"Do you think that light could have something to do with a life force that runs throughout the cosmos?"

"I guess it's possible," I muttered.

I thought back to a program I had heard the other day on the radio. A nuclear physicist was being interviewed by a CBC Radio host who was having as much trouble following his concept as I was. The man was trying to draw some sort of analogy for that soul force. He had related it to light—how light was a part of everything and nothing. He went on and on about the things that we thought were solid being mostly nothing—minuscule particles—protons, neutrons, and electrons whirling in an ocean of space. It was as though all matter were an illusion, a trick of light itself.

"Have you ever heard of Edgar Cayce?" the swami asked.

Her voice snapped me back to the moment. I had just been wrestling with the concept that if all matter were an illusion, how could anything I was experiencing now be real?

"Rita! Rita, could you find a copy of *There Is a River* for Dr. Perrin to take with him, and also the book about Yogananda Paramahansa."

The sudden realization that Dr. Perrin was leaving, going back to his own situation, struck me full force. It was as though the last few hours had only been a respite from reality. The good doctor now had to go back and face the music.

My mind was whirling. What an opera this last year would make—I could just picture the characters strutting about the stage, howling in Italian at the top of their lungs. Unrequited love, betrayal by a best friend, the death of a son—it was all there. Beethoven would have had a field day with this plot!

I watched the opera unfold. It is spring; everything is sprouting to life. The star dances through a newly plowed field. We can see dead cows stacked in a black rotting mound. Legs stick out here, heads there. A coyote runs off; crows pick at eyeballs and protruding rectums. The hero is on his knees before a beautiful young maiden. He belts out his melancholic verse as a pickup truck flies through the air. Bodies are strewn about. The curtain falls with our character wailing beside his son's coffin.

How could I possibly face John? How could I look into his eyes knowing that I was responsible for his brother's death, knowing that had I minded my own business, he would right this moment be on a farm in southern Alberta?

A sob erupted with such force that it took even the swami by surprise. I raised my hand to my face in an attempt to hide from her gaze. My sobbing subsided, and a long period of silence followed. When I finally looked toward Swami Radha, she was sitting with her eyes closed. The palms of her hands were face up, resting in her lap. I was overcome by a sense of peace as I stared at her. She was so relaxed. She had a look of utter tranquillity on her face.

"Would you be open to learning a few techniques for controlling your emotions, David?"

I flushed and quickly looked away from her. Had she known all along that I had been sitting here watching her? Could swamis see with their eyes closed?

"Yes," I managed to mumble in reply. "I would."

"Do you see that idol over there?" She pointed to a towering brass figure that I recognized as the Buddha.

"Yes."

"The Buddha teaches us that in order to be happy, in order to experience true joy, we have to be free. I'm not talking about freedom from a physical prison, or even political freedom. I'm referring to freedom from things like anger and jealousy and despair." She paused and looked into the distance for a moment before beginning again in a resolute tone. "If you look at your own situation right this very moment, do you feel in danger?"

I shook my head passively. She took a deep breath and continued. "If you look at this very moment, is there anything so bad about it that you can't go on?"

I took stock of how I felt and where I was this very moment and again shook my head.

"Then you will acknowledge that your pain is either in your past or somewhere far off in an uncertain future?"

I reluctantly nodded. Swami Radha was silent for a moment. Although she said nothing, she still seemed to be conveying an important message.

"Those of us who follow the yogic path work to keep ourselves in the now. There's no question that there will be times in your life when you'll experience pain, but by staying in the moment you rob your mind of an opportunity to prolong your suffering. Thinking has become a disease. Your mind wants nothing more than to keep you enslaved to a stream of incessant thoughts."

I was trying to follow her line of thinking. I certainly knew all about that stream of thoughts.

"I can't teach you all there is to know about the yogic path in an afternoon, David. I've been studying for thirty years and am still gaining insights on a daily basis. But I can share a few things with you that may make the next few weeks a little easier to endure."

I waited with anticipation—a hope that somewhere in all this pain was some meaning.

"Mind can be controlled by using your breath. Just close your eyes and sit as I was a moment ago." She smiled at the look of surprise on my face. She knew that I had been watching her. "Relax your body. Lean against the sofa so that your back is supported." Her voice took on an almost hypnotic tone as she continued. "Breathe in to the count of four and out to the count of four …Focus on the tip of your nostrils…Feel the air going in and the air going out. Follow it all the way down to your lungs if you can…If you find thoughts invade, then say 'in-n-n' and 'ou-u-u-t' with your breath or repeat 'ham' on the breath in and 'sa' on the breath out. Haammm, ssaaa, haammm, ssaaa."

After a few minutes, I peeked across the room. There she was—silent and serene, her palms facing the heavens as though collecting energy from the universe.

Half an hour later she spoke. "Very good, David." I had begun to squirm and it must have been obvious to her that I had reached the end of my concentration span. I opened my eyes, took a deep breath, and rotated my neck. "Do you see how good it feels to have just a few moments in the now?"

I nodded.

"Have you ever heard of *mantra*?"

"No," I said, again tipping my head to try and release some of the tension in my neck.

"Mantras are words of power that are formulations of devotion to different aspects of the Divine. They've been passed down for centuries. By repeating these powerful words over and over, and by focusing on both their sound and their vibration, they will have an effect on your mind. They become a focal point for concentration and lead to a state of meditation. Just as vibrations can affect the water in a glass, so also can they stir the subconscious mind. But just remember that emotions are meant to be controlled, not done away with."

I sighed deeply. From my point of view, it all seemed so hopeless. It was as if the swami had read my mind.

"You are a very angry man right now. I know that it seems the entire world is against you—that there is nothing but pain and suffering. You have to realize that the Divine works in wondrous ways. Nothing happens by accident. You have attracted these painful situations to you because you were not prepared to listen to Divine Mother's voice. You chose the circumstances that you were born into to best teach you the lessons you needed to learn. Unless you start listening to her, Divine Mother will send you the same lessons over and over until you finally understand."

I stared at the swami in disbelief. Was I going to be a harbinger of death with people around me dropping like flies? Would I always be the source of pain and suffering to those I loved? Would I have to live this way life after life after life?

"Don't look so troubled, David. Things are unfolding as they were meant to. You were not brought here by accident. You came under Divine Mother's guidance." Swami Radha smiled softly. "Enough for now—just remember that once you recognize her in your life, she'll never take no for an answer."

I gave the woman a sheepish grin. I couldn't help but feel that I had just been forewarned.

"Rita! The good doctor is going to do some mantra in the hall bedroom. Could you make certain there are a couple of chairs for us?"

We were seated side by side in a small room near the entrance to the house. I was a bit nervous with this new departure.

"Shiva is the aspect of the Divine for overcoming obstacles,"

Swami Radha said matter-of-factly. "I think we'll call upon him to ask for assistance. Why don't you just sing along with me?"

"Sing? I'm sorry, but I don't sing." I laughed nervously. "I've never been able to sing."

"Come on, this is very simple...Just join me." She closed her eyes, crossed her ankles, and put her hands into the position that I had seen them in earlier. She began slowly, pronouncing each syllable clearly with a varying intensity. "Om-na-mah-si-va-ya, Om namah sivaya, Om namah sivaya, Om namah sivaya."

I listened to her beautiful voice for over a minute before I finally made a nervous attempt to clear my throat. At first, I just repeated the words. It seemed too much to ask to actually try to sing them. I repeated them a dozen times.

"Now put your heart into it, David. You told me you had grief for Brian—that you loved him. Let me hear that pain."

"Om namah sivaya, Om namah sivaya, Om namah sivaya, Om namah sivaya."

"Give your pain to Shiva," Swami Radha interjected. "Let him take it from you."

"Om namah sivaya! Om namah sivaya! Om namah..." I was soon belting out the mantra and drowning the sweet voice that was acting as my template. My voice cracked constantly on the higher notes; tears streamed down my face. I bellowed on.

It was getting dark before I left the ashram. My mind was still reeling. I knew it was time for some changes in my life.

I talked with Mom and Dad when I went back to pick up Lug, touching on the obvious points about Brian and the struggles I was having with practice. Somehow I felt that I owed them more. Was there any possible way they could understand what a roller-coaster ride I was on? How I wished now that the avenues for better communication between us had been built and maintained earlier in life.

I drove as if in a trance on the way back to Creston. It was with a start that I came upon the sign announcing Twin Bays. I glanced down the hill in an accusatory fashion—had the boy at least enjoyed his last moments here?

Tension built as I headed down the steep hill into the Sirdar crossing. Had Brian even the slightest premonition of the danger he was in as he flew by this tiny burg? I slowed as I covered the next few miles searching for skid marks—peering over the steep embankment for signs of skinned trees or broken shrubs.

I drove on, certain that each corner would be revealed as the one to have claimed the boy's life. I was almost to Wynndel before I admitted that I had passed it by. How could I have missed it? How could a site of such importance go unmarked? The roadway blurred.

"Om namah sivaya! Om namah sivaya! Om namah sivaya! Om namah sivaya!"

The Funeral

Pulling into the parking lot, I turned off the ignition and stared up at the dilapidated old building that had served as home for the clinic. My eyes focused on a few areas on the north corner. The layer of white paint was streaky and the grey still showed through. The boys and I had gotten a bit lax with our painting back there— just ran out of steam. I could still visualize the pair of them hanging over the edge of the ridgecap with their rollers, white paint smeared from their running shoes to the tops of their heads. They never did tell me what had started that paint fight three long years before.

Lug swatted me with his paw and nuzzled my shoulder. He was anxious to check out his territory. I opened the door and he bounded over me. Following after him, I trudged along the side of the clinic to Canyon Street and gingerly poked my head around the corner of the building. The last thing I wanted was to meet a friend or client who wanted to chat. I hated to even think of the terrible shambles my life was in—and I certainly didn't want to discuss it with someone else.

The rickety door at the bottom of the stairwell pushed in with a rattle and scraped across the surface of the warped grey boards that comprised the landing. Lug zipped past me and galloped to the top deck. Turning to watch me, he grinned and wagged his tail exuberantly. How I wished I could share some of his spark, exhibit even a bit of his enthusiasm. No matter what the circumstances, the dog lived in the moment—why, he even loved returning to this old dump.

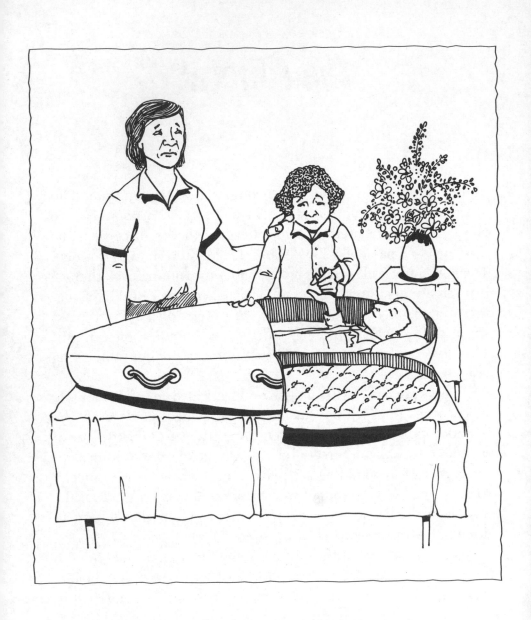

But he was totally unaware that I was dreading the thought of meeting John. Lug would proceed with his usual growling and grumping in pretense of defending his territory—then he would lick the boy half to death.

I put the key in the lock and rattled the handle up and down until the mechanism gave way with a clunk. I followed Lug into the apartment and wandered into the living room. Surely I could think of something meaningful that needed doing. The telephone rang. I ran to get it before realizing that it was no longer my job to answer it. Not only was I not on call, but I wasn't even part of the practice anymore.

I checked out the spare room. The bed was neatly made and nowhere was there any evidence that Marcie and Cory had even been there. They hadn't wasted any time in getting out. I wondered if they would be happier living with Doris. How quickly things changed—how slowly I wanted to adjust.

Om namah sivaya, Om namah sivaya. I struggled with tears, woeful notions, and the silent repetition of the mantra all in the same moment. *Get away, thoughts. Leave me alone!* Swami Radha had cautioned me not to battle with the wayward snippets that traipsed through my mind. Just recognize them, she said, and release them. What a tall order that was! Sort of like releasing a bee into the midst of its swarm and hoping that it wouldn't come back to bother me.

I had been noticing my mental antics on the way into town and couldn't believe the unrelenting jumble. It was as if someone had taken frames from each of a hundred movies and played them over and over in different sequences and combinations.

Slowing my breath, I followed the air into my lungs, feeling my chest rise and fall. I finally picked up the receiver. June Miller, owner of Creston Taxi, was now acting as an answering service. She was taking a message from John Partington about the condition of a downer cow that Cory had treated. "Tell him she's no better," the dairyman reiterated as he hung up.

My mind was whirling as I was assailed by the irritating sound of the dial tone. I wondered if Cory had gotten a blood sample to send to the lab. Had he given any thought to the possibility that selenium and phosphorus levels might have something to do with the fact that the cow couldn't stand up?

I shook my head as I realized that I hadn't begun to let go of the affairs of the clinic. I just had to back off and hope that Cory would work things out on his own. *Close your eyes, big fella ...Breathe deeply. Count to four. Haaammm, sssaaa. Haammm, sssaaa. Haaammm, sssaaa.*

I dialled Martha's number and waited uncomfortably as it buzzed. She answered on the third ring.

"Hello, Martha. Is he there?"

"I'm sorry, Dave, he's not. I'm surprised you haven't heard from him. He called and asked for you several times at the clinic…It's so hard to get hold of you now that you aren't there alone."

"I know…I'm sorry about that." It was strange that I had never given thought to getting a private number—Dave and Creston Veterinary Hospital had always been one and the same in my mind. "How has he been doing?"

"He's taking it hard," said Martha. "But you know John…That boy has a special steel about him. He's up at the funeral parlour right now picking out a coffin."

"Oh God," I moaned. Tears flooded my eyes at the very thought of John wandering alone into the funeral home. What business had he even being there at his age? It was obscene for an eighteen-year-old boy to be choosing a coffin for his younger brother.

"I better get up there," I said uncertainly.

"He wanted you there with him," Martha added. "He said it was like the three of you were brothers. Just to warn you…the boy asked if I would mind terribly if he stayed with you tonight."

"Thanks, Martha." I hung up the receiver, closed my eyes, and focused on the tip of my nose. *Haammm, sssaaa. Haammm, sssaaa.*

I pushed the buzzer on the side of the yellow stucco building. George Oliver was at the door within minutes.

"Hello, Dave." The gentle, grey-haired man trained compassionate eyes on mine. Dressed in his customary black suit and muted grey tie, his shoulders stooped more than I had ever noticed previously—he seemed burdened by the weight of the world. I wondered at having to prepare two sixteen-year-olds for burial. How had he endured all these years as the town's mortician? He gave me an apologetic smile and rested his hand on my forearm. "I'm so sorry. John told me you were close to them both. The boy's been expecting you."

Although not many people were anxious to use George's services, he was one of the town's most popular citizens. The man was always so genuine, so prepared to help others without the slightest thought to their status in the community. Not once since I'd met him had I ever heard him make a nasty comment about another person.

"He's with Brian now," George said quietly. "This is his second session."

I nodded and followed the man to the viewing parlour. John turned as we walked into the room. He was so out of place in this chamber of death—this innocent, baby-faced boy with long frizzy hair. Turning away from the coffin, he let go of his brother's hand. Silently, he took a step in my direction, then halted. His eyes brimmed with tears.

I focused on his face and struggled to keep from looking at the coffin. How could this be happening?

"I'm so sorry, John."

The boy shook his head and half turned toward his brother. "I keep talking to him, Dave, hoping that he can hear me somehow. I had so many things I wanted to tell him...I don't think he ever knew how important he was to me."

"I know, John...I know."

"When we were kids, we did everything together. I thought we'd be able to talk about all the things we went through later—

you know, when we were old men and had good lives. Now, he's lying here in a box and I don't even know if he can hear me."

I rested my arm on the boy's shoulder and for the first time allowed myself to peer into the coffin. Brian was dressed in a white shirt and tie. The only time I recalled seeing him with one of those infernal things wrapped around his neck was at John's graduation. He had wriggled and squirmed and complained about it constantly. I hated to see him burdened with it now. Oh God, he looked so different—his face swollen, misshapen—pale even with all that makeup.

John lifted his brother's hand again and cupped it between his. "Do you think it's all right to be talking to him, Dave? We used to confide in each other about everything. I was just telling him about this girl I met. Brian woulda liked Lydia…you would, too. She's pretty neat."

I closed my eyes tightly and fought back the tears. I had to keep my cool. For once, I had to be strong.

"You tell him everything, John. I think he's listening." The aching in my throat increased exponentially. The pressure of tears built until I was certain I would explode.

"I picked out the best coffin they have. It's all wood—mahogany. I want Brian to have the best. We always had stuff that was left over from other people—stuff that was sort of just good enough."

I stood behind the boy as he studied his brother's lifeless form. How I wanted to take John in my arms and hug him—hug him for all the opportunities that I had missed in the past, hug him for all the times I had failed his brother. What was stopping me?

"Do you think he suffered, Dave?"

"I guess we'll never know, John. All we can do is hope that he didn't—hope that it was quick."

"You know, Brian hardly ever complained. I think back on all those nights in Calgary when we went to bed hungry, and all the times when we'd sit up and listen to Mom's parties. We used to peek out through a crack in the door to see what was going on."

The boy paused and squeezed Brian's hand as if hoping for a response. "Some nights guys would open our door and come crashing in…Mom would yell at them. We'd lie there in the dark with our eyes closed and our hearts pounding—pretending we were asleep. We'd breathe deeply—hoping they'd go away and leave us alone."

I grasped his shoulder and he stopped talking briefly as if I had wakened him from a dream.

"We always wondered who was going to be there when we woke up in the morning…which of the guys would be wrapped around the can passed out when we went for a pee. We always hoped there'd be some chips or pop left for us. Sometimes there was cold pizza or leftover Chinese food for breakfast."

The back of John's head blurred as tears flooded my eyes. I wanted so much to go back to that apartment and protect those boys—to erase all their misery and heal all their wounds. How could such beautiful boys be burdened with so much pain? Why was life so unfair? Why could I not take the boy in my arms this very moment and tell him that things were going to be all right?

"Have you eaten today, John?"

"Martha made me a sandwich when I got here." He released Brian's hand and straightened the ridiculous tie. "I haven't been very hungry, to be honest."

"Let's go for supper."

John looked helplessly at the coffin. "I don't want to leave him."

"I know, John. You were always there for him when he was alive, too. You know that…He knows that. I wish there was something that we could change right now, but I just don't know what it is."

His face contorted and he burst into tears. "Some day, years from now…I'll want to hold him, Dave. I'll want so much to see his face again, and I won't be able to."

I squeezed his shoulder, wiped away the tears that trickled down my face.

"Dave…" John hesitated. "This sounds stupid…but…Brian hated the dark. I remember when we were younger I locked him in a big trunk that Mom had. He screamed and screamed until we got it open." The boy stopped, lost in thought.

I left the room in search of George. He was slumped in a swivel chair behind a big oak desk in his office. I wondered if he had slept at all the previous night.

"George?"

His eyes snapped open. He smiled sheepishly and rotated his chair to face in my direction.

"Sorry to bother you, George, but I have a question."

"What is it, Dave?" He suppressed a yawn and rubbed at his eyes with the back of his hand.

"This may sound like a strange question, but where do you store the bodies? Do you have a cooler room or something?"

I felt stupid—as if I was prying into a business that wasn't my own. I knew how people felt the first time they showed up at my veterinary hospital and stared in wonderment at all the stainless gadgets, not having an inkling of what they were for. It was the same here—I hadn't a clue how George carried out the day-to-day operation of his business.

"I'm not sure I understand what you mean, Dave."

"I'm sorry, but John hates the thought of closing the lid on his brother's coffin. Brian was always afraid of confinement—a bit claustrophobic, I guess. Is there some way the boy can be stored so that John won't be fretting?"

"Certainly, Dave. As a matter of fact, we can leave him right where he is for now. Once I've done the embalming, the body doesn't need to be in a cooler. I can leave him there with the coffin open."

"Thank you, George. John will feel much better about that."

"I don't know what we'll do about tomorrow, though. I don't

know of a minister who would do a service with an open coffin—
I'm sure Vanderlie won't be interested. He was the only one I could
get on such short notice—John wanted the service tomorrow."

"We can deal with that in the morning. I'll see if I can get John
to go home with me right now. I'm sure he'll feel a bit less apprehensive…You look as if you could use some sleep."

George smiled acceptingly. I recognized the symptoms of a
sleepless night. I had done twenty-four-hour stretches often
enough myself to understand how the man was feeling.

John picked absently at the stack of French fries that remained on
his plate. He had pretty much demolished the hamburger, but the
fries and coleslaw were heading back to the kitchen.

"You ready to go?"

The boy nodded half-heartedly. Picking up the bill, I headed
for the till. I waited as the elderly couple in front of us paid for
their meal and tottered out to the street. John drifted after them as
I waited for the waitress to ring up our bill.

"He sure looks like a woebegone waif tonight." Shirley was our
favourite waitress. She had served us dozens of times over the
years. "I'm so sorry to hear about his brother."

I nodded and passed her a twenty-dollar bill. My eyes brimmed
with tears as she mechanically passed me my change.

"They seemed like such nice boys," she murmured almost
to herself.

John and I wandered side by side up the street toward the
office. The silence was unbearable—I was so used to his rattling
on about his daily adventures. It was painful to see him so subdued. We clumped up the stairs to the landing. Lug whined anxiously inside as I fiddled with the key in the lock. For the most
part, I secured the door more to protect people from him than to
keep someone from stealing anything. Not many folks were anxious to try the door when he was barking and slavering noisily on
the other side of it. The moment I swung it open, he danced

around excitedly, licking madly at John's hands, and jumping up on us in alternate fashion.

"Settle down, boy. Settle down."

"Hey there, fella, I missed you, too."

John knelt next to the big goof and smiled unwittingly as the dog's tongue swabbed his face. Critters had such an amazing ability to get beyond people's defences—to force them openly into moments of joy.

I threw myself full-length onto the stuffed cushion on the living room carpet. John slumped into the recliner and rested his head against the support. Taking a deep breath, he released an audible sigh. Lug nestled his head in the boy's lap and looked knowingly up at him.

"How are things going with your apprenticeship, John?"

"Good, really…I like sheet-metal work and it looks like it'll be easy to get a job when I'm done."

"That's great—there's nothing more important than being happy with what you're doing. A guy spends a lot of time working, and it can make life pretty difficult to endure if there's no enjoyment in it."

"Yeah, and…" John stopped mid-sentence. There was a moment of uncomfortable silence. "It's just not fair, Dave."

"I know, John. Nothing's been fair for either of you for as long as I've known you. You've been dealt some pretty nasty cards."

John gazed absently at a ceiling tile that undoubtedly showed his future carefully mapped out before him. He gradually stopped stroking Lug's head. As if sensing the boy's detachment, the dog rambled over to collapse in a heap next to me. Stretching his head back, he rested it next to my thigh within easy reach of an idle hand.

"I feel so responsible for what happened to him, John. I was sulking about my own problems and let the boy get into trouble. If I'd been here or if I'd just minded my own business and left him in Alberta, none of this would have happened."

"You didn't even know when he was coming," John interjected. "Martha told me Brian wanted to surprise you. It's more my fault than yours. That's all I've been thinking since I found out he got killed…If I had paid more attention to what was going on, he'd have come to Calgary instead. He wouldn't have been so unhappy…You know I only went down to see him once in all that time he was on the farm, and they wouldn't let him come into the city. I shoulda known better than to let him go to Taber."

"I guess all that's in the past now, John. There are so many things that would have made a difference if only we'd known. I guess not many people would have accidents if everyone could see into the future. Of all the kids to die because of alcohol, though…Had Brian ever been drunk in his life?"

John wagged his head mechanically. "Not that I know of…We drained a few of Mom's bottles when we were younger and got a bit of a buzz on. But I sure don't remember him ever really drinking. We hated what it did to Mom. Wouldn't you know—all those years of her boozing and nothing terrible ever happened. Now this, when Brian was just along for the ride. Who knows if he had anything to drink? I guess it really doesn't matter."

He again stared vacantly at the ceiling while I watched him and toyed absently with Lug's floppy ear. I let it fall limply to the side of his head. The dog snoozed on, totally oblivious to my tinkering. I got up and put on a Neil Diamond record. I was already reclining on the cushion again when the singer started belting out "Love on the Rocks." I snorted. Where else could love possibly be?

"I think I'm going to bed, Dave. I'm real tired…I never got any sleep last night."

I turned the volume of the record player down. "The bed's made up for you."

"Thanks." He headed to the bathroom.

The record was soon finished and I was off to bed myself. I felt so deep-down weary, so emotionally drained. I was halfway across the living room when I heard it. I stopped and listened. The sound was unmistakeable. John was sobbing in his room. I stood at the door for several minutes trying to build the courage to knock.

"John," I called timidly. I opened the door and ventured in.

"Oh, Dave, I miss him so much. He's lying in that box."

I sat on the edge of the bed. Only John's head stuck out from beneath the covers. His face buried in the pillow, he wept uncontrollably. His body was wracked by wave after wave of sobbing. All I could do was rest my hand on his shoulder. Why couldn't I give the boy the support he needed? Why did I have to be such a cold son of a bitch?

"I know how you feel, John. I miss him, too."

"He's all alone, Dave. I shoulda stayed with him."

"We have to believe that he's not alone anymore, John. You know that there was more to Brian than is lying up there in that box. There has to be a part of him that nothing can destroy."

I draped my arm over John and let the tears flow. *Please, Lord…may what I said be true. May that beautiful boy's spirit be somewhere safe. May we someday meet again.*

Within a half hour we had both cried ourselves out. John's breathing was deep and rhythmic. He looked relaxed—thank God for sleep. I studied his face. There was no doubt about it—I loved the boy. He was family.

The organ droned as we waited for the proceedings to begin. I sat to the left of John. Martha sat on his right holding his hand. I was worried about the service. The minister had arrived a few minutes before we had taken our seats, and when George introduced him to me, he struck me as a pompous ass. I was hoping that he would rise above himself for this occasion.

The chapel of the funeral home rapidly filled to overflowing. Brian and John had touched so many people in their few short years in our midst. I had never seen so many young faces in a place of worship before. The casket, which stood closed at the front of the room, was covered with flowers. John had requested that it remain open as long as possible. Although the boy didn't say more about it to me, the minister must not have been amenable to the suggestion.

John looked around apprehensively. I could see he was struggling to retain his composure. He had spent an hour in the early morning going over details of his family's life with the minister. I was relieved when the man finally cleared his throat and began his oration. It gave us something to focus on other than our pain. With the beginning of the Lord's Prayer, I rested my hand on John's arm and squeezed gently. We mumbled our way through it and held back our tears. I hoped we would both be able to maintain our composure.

From the outset of the service, I grew more uneasy. My first impression of the churchman had obviously been right. He had been ranting for twenty minutes now and hadn't mentioned Brian's name once. I glanced to my right. John's face was pale and tense—poker straight. I glared at the minister with the hopes of catching his attention, but to no avail. He was focused on all those young faces in the chairs behind us. Froth accumulated in the corner of his mouth. Occasionally, during moments of intensity, he projected sprays of spittle. His face was red and the veins at his temples bulged as he assailed the youths. He went on and on about the "grim reaper," threatening the congregation with his appearance when they were least expecting him.

"Brian didn't expect him!" he hollered. "Was he ready?"

My entire body tensed. It was all I could do to remain seated, to keep from getting up and kicking this man's sorry ass onto the street where he belonged. I glanced at John. His eyes were closed, his head bowed.

I was a total wreck by the time the loudspeakers came to life with the spiritual, "He's Got the Whole World in His Hands." The moment John heard it, his composure cracked and he burst into tears. He wanted them to play the song—it had been a family favourite that he and Brian had sung with their mother in happier days. The soothing music seemed out of place after listening to the fool hurtling fire and brimstone at his captive audience. George and his assistant, Norman, walked solemnly to the coffin. A group of teens, looking uncomfortable in formal clothes, rose on signal and stepped forward to serve as pallbearers. Their complexions were ashen, their eyes downcast. John wept on.

The funeral procession to the cemetery snaked its way down the side street and onto Canyon. John and I sat in the back seat of the lead car. A train of vehicles with their lights on stretched as far back as the eye could see. A tragedy like this hit close to the heart of a sleepy little town like Creston.

John's eyes met mine. It was as if we could read each other's minds. Neither of us could believe that when this ordeal was over, Brian's life would be nothing more than a memory. I reached over and took his hand. Tears welled in our eyes, and we turned to focus on the road ahead.

The hearse backed up to a pile of dirt just above a little side road. I approached the graveside and looked out over the valley—Brian certainly had a nice view.

I stood close to John as George supervised the positioning of the coffin. The minister droned on in front of a sea of faces. His presentation was thankfully short and succinct. John and I remained until all the people at the burial had nodded their condolences and drifted away.

We stood there for twenty minutes contemplating that fancy mahogany box. Finally George came over and mumbled to John in his practised muted voice. The boy plucked a white carnation from one of the bouquets on the top of the coffin, and George and Norman lowered it into the ground.

John threw a handful of dirt on top of the magnificent wood, and I followed suit. It seemed so unfair to be hiding such beauty beneath all that dirt. How could this possibly be the end of the boy who had so inched his way into my heart?

Bald Boys Selling Flowers

I spent the morning with John before he headed off to his new life in Calgary. Most of our time together was spent in silence. Neither of us was ready to accept the fact that Brian was truly gone from our lives. When we did speak, it was invariably to wish that we had managed our affairs with him differently.

John insisted on spending his last hour in Creston at the gravesite. He now felt a connection with the mound of dirt beneath which his brother lay. He stood beside it talking away, as though he now had a reference point from which to deal with his memories. I sat on the grass at some distance, staring out over the valley below.

I wondered if I'd ever return to this meagre plot of ground. Although the final physical remains of Brian Joachim Gallagher would in fact remain beneath that mound, his spirit certainly didn't belong there. What had become of that indefinable light? Where was the spark that crackled from those big blue eyes? What had become of that smouldering glow that always appeared along with his stubborn streak?

It was late afternoon by the time I arrived at my parents' place in Riondel. I sat back on the sofa. Resting my head against the wall, I closed my eyes and allowed my thoughts to wander.

Along with all the other misery that was happening in my life, I just couldn't accept the way things had turned out with Marcie. It was bad enough that she wanted nothing more to do with me, but why did Cory have to fall for her? I wasn't sure what upset me,

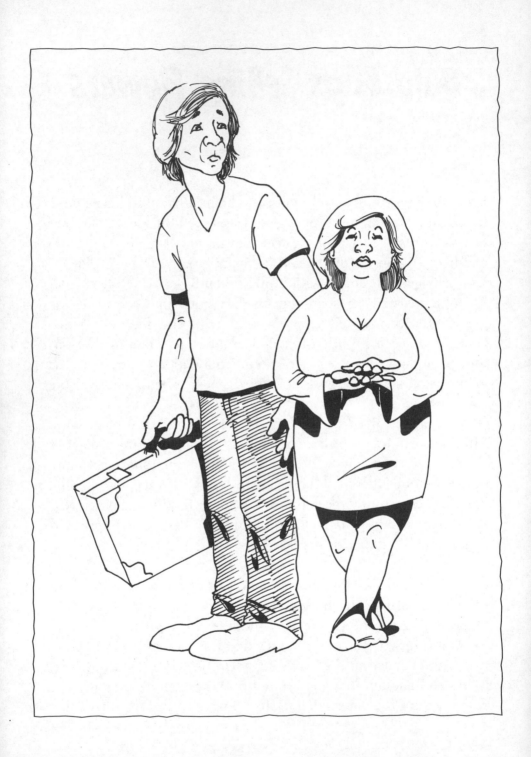

more—seeing Marcie with another man or feeling alienated from the guy I had once considered my best friend.

And then there was the issue of the boys. Why had I not been able to bring more joy to Brian's life? Why could I not be there to truly support his brother in his time of need? Would I ever learn to co-exist with other human beings? Where was God at times like this? If He really knew all the answers, why was He so reluctant to share even a few of them with a lost soul like me?

Now that I was here with Mom and Dad, would I tell them what was actually going on in my life? How much of the puzzle had they pieced together? I knew they were wondering where Marcie fit in. How was I going to break it to Dad that I was about to limp off to places unknown and give away the practice that I had struggled so hard to establish?

I sighed. Nothing was pressing on Father's mind right at the moment. He was stretched out in his easy chair, his feet up, his head lodged at an uncomfortable angle, and his mouth open wide. He snored in fits and starts. The Louis L'Amour novel he was reading remained open in his outstretched hand.

Mother bustled around in the kitchen. By the smell of it, she was preparing fried chicken. Poor Mom, she had been trying desperately to elevate my spirits. She knew there was nothing like her chicken to get me salivating.

"Marsh! Dave! Supper's ready."

Father stirred, staring at his book with bleary eyes. He held it at arm's length to imply that he'd been reading all along. I smiled and got to my feet. I was hungry—I wouldn't need to be called a second time.

We ate in silence aside from the niceties of "Pass this" and "Pass that." Lug sat at my side, drooling as he watched the pile of chicken bones build on the side of my plate. I had funnelled him pieces of skin and bits of the cartilaginous portions from the ends of bones, so that every time I moved he shifted hopefully in my direction.

"Do you think you could look after Lug for me for a couple of weeks?" I asked.

"No problem," Father answered. "You going to take a bit of a holiday without him?"

"I'm thinking of spending a few weeks at the ashram, just up the lake."

My mother's face fell. I recognized the look of apprehension that I had grown so used to during my years growing up in Casino.

"Are you sure you want to go down there, Dave?" she asked. "The neighbours have told us some pretty strange stories about that place. Aren't they the same outfit as those bald-headed boys they show pictures of selling flowers at airports and street corners?"

"No, Mom, they're not the same."

"They had a news special on those kids just the other day, didn't they, Marsh? You remember. They were talking about how their handlers took all their stuff away—even their clothes. They shaved their hair and gave them funny-looking outfits to wear and made them sell flowers to try and earn enough money to feed themselves."

I shifted in my seat and looked in desperation at my father for support. "They're not the same, Mom!" I snapped.

Excusing myself from the table, I stomped to the door. My face was flushed; Mother had hit that spot one more time. If I had learned anything over the years, it was to get away from her before I exploded. A tirade right now was the last thing anyone needed, and once Mom got off on a tangent, there would be no quick way of changing her direction.

"Come on, Lug. Let's go for a walk."

My eyes were brimming with tears as I headed down the alley to the main thoroughfare. Within a few blocks, Hedley Street ran into Eastman Avenue. Eastman was continuous with the road that meandered for miles north along Kootenay Lake. I had in mind a trek to where Tam O'Shanter Creek dumped into the main body. Lug loved nothing better than to get out in the boonies and rummage around for something to excite his olfactory senses. We stopped on a little stretch of beach before the boat launch. The dog waded into water up to his belly, lapping as he went.

"Hey! You're going to get us in even more trouble with Grandma. You know she doesn't like it when you come back wet."

I grabbed a stick from the beach and tossed it twenty feet in front of him. He splashed out after it. As if to please Grandma even more, he ducked his head completely beneath the surface. His mouth came up gnashing ruthlessly at the hapless piece of wood. Whining all the way to shore, he presented it for me to throw again. Oh, for a transfusion of some of his energy.

It was almost dark by the time we got back to the house. Lug's tongue was hanging as he puffed his way along. His coat had long since dried and he easily endured Grandma's scrutiny.

"Where have you been all this time?" she asked.

"We walked down to Tam O'Shanter Creek."

"Oh my, that's a long way. No wonder the poor dog looks so tired."

"When are you planning on going down there?" Father asked, putting an unusual emphasis on the word "there."

"Tomorrow morning," I replied.

I was in no hurry as I drove down the road to the ashram. If it hadn't been for the set of circumstances surrounding Brian's death, this would be the last place on earth that I would consider going. Even now, I argued the merits of hiking into Meachen Lake instead. After all, what did I really know about this offbeat establishment?

There was a part of me that shared my mother's deep foreboding, that made me worry about letting someone I knew little about tinker with my mind. Maybe I would find myself selling flowers in some far-off airport. My mind flashed immediately to the strange little depression in the back of my head—the hollow that Father used to delight in exposing when he cut my hair. I glanced in the car mirror—at the hair that hung over my ears. No way would anybody shave me bald!

I pulled up in front of the bookstore and walked in, displaying what I hoped was a casual attitude.

"Hello, Dr. Perrin." It was the same woman who had greeted me the last time around.

"Hello," I responded.

"Are you here for a bit of a stay? Swami Radha told us you'd likely be joining us for a while."

I hesitated, thinking once more about the panoramic view from the campsite on the shores of Meachen Lake, picturing the snow-capped peak of Haystack Mountain.

"Yes…I'm here to check in."

Lugging my suitcase, I followed my guide up a steep set of stairs to a bench a hundred feet above the parking lot. By the look of this woman's lean figure, she must have tackled this ascent frequently. I was struggling to control my breath and keep from huffing. At the landing, we followed a concrete walkway toward the larger of two Panabode buildings. Constructed of milled cedar logs, it appeared to have been recently completed.

As we passed in front of a long set of windows, I noted with interest what was obviously a yoga class in progress. Participants floated around the perimeter of the room, making circular patterns with their hands as if lifting some invisible matter.

We entered through the small foyer in the centre of the building. My guide held the door open as I struggled through with my suitcase, then stopped short and removed her shoes.

"Your room is on the second floor."

Flicking off my right shoe with the toe of my left, I fired it onto one of the trays by the door. I was working the other shoe off when a stout, middle-aged woman emerged from the classroom. Moving in slow motion, she passed between us. Her eyes half closed and her open hands elevated, she deliberately placed one foot in front of the other.

"I am focusing from my centre," she affirmed in a whisper. "I am focusing from my centre."

My guide headed through the alcove and up the stairs. I stood staring as the woman disappeared down a hallway.

Oh Lord, what had I gotten myself into?

My accommodation was more than adequate. For the moment, I'd be alone in a spacious double room. The planed surface of the cedar logs gave the area a muted, rustic touch. A pair of desks was situated on the far wall beneath a large window. Light streamed through to make the room bright and cheery. I threw myself onto the bed to try out the springs and landed with a resounding thud. Lifting the mattress, I confirmed what I had already suspected—there were no springs. Two inches of foam would separate my body from a board platform.

I began pacing—just as Lug did when he was ready for his walk. What was I to do with myself? Opening my suitcase, I slipped a few shirts on hangers and stashed them in the closet. I wondered if I'd ever be able to get into the flow of things here—right at that moment, I felt so out of place. My guide had explained how to find Main House, the building where meals would be served. Lunch would be at 12:30. I was to be informed then when I'd be able to see Swami Radha.

I shuffled about my room. Absently plucking the Yogananda book that the swami had given me from my suitcase, I opened it to chapter one. I got no further than the first paragraph, then tossed it on the desk. I just didn't feel like reading. Wandering into the hall, I made my way down the stairs and sat in the foyer long enough to slip on my shoes.

Outside on the sidewalk, I peered through the window into the classroom. I felt like a voyeur. The class was still in progress. Students sat motionlessly on the floor with their legs crossed.

Nothing appeared to be going on. I wondered if they were in meditation. There was so much about this place I just didn't understand.

For several minutes, I stood on the top step of the landing and gazed. From there, the lake lay like a huge silver plain beckoning to be explored. I plunked my way down the steps, passed the bookstore, and continued downhill toward an old wooden building with a sign that identified itself as Main House. A blue jay landed in the apple tree above me. Hurling insults in my direction, he cocked his head and gawked down at me. I stopped to watch him hop from branch to branch, then descended a set of stone stairs. A sign informed me I had arrived at the Beach Prayer House. Rounding the corner of the cedar-shake building, I wandered onto a strip of grass that parallelled the beach.

The stones that bordered the water were smooth and similar to one another in size and shape; from a distance only their colour set them apart. I marvelled at their uniformity as they ground beneath the soles of my sneakers. Did this place do that to everything that was exposed to it? Would it knock the rough edges off me as well? Make me more like other people?

Picking up one of the stones, I ran my fingers over its velvety surface. I wondered how many years of abrasion it had taken to bring it to that perfect state. I hurled it in the direction of the lake, where it landed with a barely audible plunk a few feet from shore. Fifty yards down the beach was a massive rock outcropping. I gravitated toward it. Worn smooth by years of pounding water and grinding stones, it looked as if it had been honed as a throne just for me. What a peaceful spot. I settled myself on the cool granite surface and stared dreamily across the shimmering water.

There was not a cloud in sight and not a breath of wind; the water glistened with hardly a ripple. Sun glinted on a windshield miles away on the opposite shore. I watched as a car inched its way along the winding highway toward an assortment of buildings that I knew to be Ainsworth Hot Springs. I suddenly wished that

276

I was over there reclining in the steaming waters. Why was it that no matter where I was of late, I always wanted to be some-where else?

I took a deep breath and tried to push away my worries. I felt so tired, depleted of energy. How had I allowed my life to veer so out of control? Would I ever be able to regain some semblance of order?

The ringing of a bell caught my attention. I glanced at my watch. It was 12:30. Taking a final look across the water, I rose from my throne, stretched, and massaged a butt that had grown numb from sitting so long on the cool, hard surface. I made my way up the stairs to the old frame building and stood apprehen-sively near the entrance. Other than the clatter and scraping of metal utensils on plates, the room was silent. Two women rounded the corner of the building behind me. I took a deep breath, opened the screen door, and timidly stepped inside.

In the cloistered environment, four long tables were pressed against the west wall; benches on either side of them were filled with people. The two women squeezed past me and made their way to the farthest table. Heads turned. I was aware of the fact that many eyes were evaluating the newcomer who had just ducked through the entrance door. I was self-consciously surveying the room when Ron stood up and motioned me to the seat beside him.

"Hi, Ron," I said enthusiastically.

He smiled and pointed to his sealed lips. I noticed that no one else in the room was talking. Stepping over the bench with my right leg, I struggled to get my left into the tiny slot allotted me. I wobbled uneasily, almost toppling onto the woman sitting on the other side of me, and landed on the seat with an unceremonious clatter.

I closed my eyes, took a deep breath, and waited until the tit-tering had died down. From now on, I'd be here early enough to pick a spot at the end of a bench. When I opened my eyes, Ron was holding a bowl of steaming rice in front of me. I took it and deposited a scoop on my plate. Someone from the opposite side of the table passed a bowl with curried vegetables. I buried the rice with several full ladles, then picked up my fork and began mixing everything together. I stared at the concoction, trying to identify what I was about to eat. There was definitely no meat. I couldn't remember ever eating curry before.

I dug in—not bad—certainly not what I was used to, but not bad. I had wolfed down half of my portion when I looked around the table at the other diners. All were eating as if in slow motion; they chewed slowly and deliberately. I stopped—I had been shovelling in two or three mouthfuls to one of everyone else's.

A woman entered and found a place at the adjoining table. Sitting gracefully in the middle of the bench, she carefully filled her plate, seemingly deliberating over each ladleful. I had almost finished my portion when she bowed her head, brought her hands together at her breast, and closed her eyes. It was several minutes before she picked up her fork and began to eat.

After the meal, I lingered behind while the others filed away from the tables. Ron sat with me as if sensing my unease. After the last diner had placed his dirty dishes in the receptacle by the door, he spoke. "How are you managing?"

"I feel terribly out of place."

"I can appreciate that. I remember what it was like on my first day here."

"Right at the moment I'm wishing I'd gone hiking."

"Just look at this as a bit of a hike…and remember that when it's over you're going to have a beautiful view from the top."

"Usually when I go hiking, I at least know what my destination is…You know, I don't know the slightest thing about this place. My mother's sure I'll end up with a shaved head selling flowers in some far-off airport."

Ron smiled and I looked away from him to the exit. "For all I know she could be right. What is this place, anyway?"

Ron suddenly looked serious. "Well, I've been here for several

278

years and still have my hair. As you may have gathered, this is a retreat where people come to study yogic principles. Swami Radha and a handful of devotees moved here in 1963. She felt that the Kootenay Bay area had a special energy, and from what I've experienced since I've been here, I tend to agree with her. When she moved here, there was little more than this old shack of a house and a few outbuildings. We're building constantly to try and meet the needs of the people who come here."

"What's the story on the swami? Are you related to her?"

Ron smiled again. "No blood relation...I guess you could call her my spiritual mother. She has a way of playing that role with a lot of us here."

"I can understand that...There's something about her. Where's she from? She sounds German."

"She is German. Although she doesn't mention her past often, I know she was born into a wealthy family in Berlin. She was apparently quite a famous dancer and had training in business. When the Nazis rose to power, she fled to Britain. Her husband died during the war and she immigrated to Canada. She had a visionary experience that led her to her guru, Swami Sivananda."

He pointed to a picture of a rather roly-poly man with a shaved head, seated in the lotus position on a tiger skin.

"She contacted him and went to India to study with him. She was initiated in 1956 and has been a renunciate and teacher ever since. She's tried to translate the yogic traditions so that Westerners like us can relate to them. A lot of the tools that we use here at the ashram are adaptations she has made of ancient Buddhist practices."

Ron stacked up his cutlery and cup on top of his plate and stood up. "Don't worry. The discomfort you're now feeling is something that we all have known. From what Swami Radha has told us at *satsangs*, she herself struggled terribly with the radical change in direction. At least we were able to do it in our own country—she did it halfway around the world."

I was still apprehensive as I made my way to Swami Radha's house, called Many Mansions. Ron had informed me that I could see her at two o'clock. I wondered where this whole experience would lead. What would the next few weeks have in store for me?

I rang the doorbell, then stepped away. Fidgeting nervously, I retreated a few steps up the path. I surveyed the orchard and the crew that was busily working in the garden. What had brought all these other people here? The door opened.

"Hello, Rita."

"Hello, Dave…Swami Radha is expecting you."

The woman led me through the hall to the sitting room. The swami was seated at a desk, making notations in the margin of some sort of manuscript. She looked up, placed her glasses on the table, and smiled at me.

"Hello, David. How did things go for you back in Creston?"

I began hesitantly, telling her first about my encounter with John. Soon, I was pouring out the details of the past few days, rattling on about the horrendous church service the minister had presented—how he had only once used Brian's name and only then to point out that the boy had not been ready to meet his maker.

"That's the problem with many organized religions," she sighed. "All too often they try and control people's thought patterns with fear. As well-meaning as the man probably was, that type of approach makes us fearful of what might happen and leaves us constantly uncertain about the future."

The swami closed her eyes for a moment, then opened them and regarded me reflectively.

"David, if I could magically take away all the traumas that you've suffered over the last year, do you think you'd be truly happy?" She took a sip of her tea and looked at me over her cup.

"I'm not sure, but I'd like to think I'd be one heck of a lot happier than I am right now."

She settled her cup gently into its saucer and stared intently at me again.

"All too often in life, unless people make major changes, they end up facing similar problems and suffering through the same sort of pain over and over again."

I waited expectantly for her to drop the other shoe.

"Have you worked at all with the mantra and the breathing exercises that I showed you?"

I nodded.

"How do you feel right now?"

"Not bad. Maybe a bit overwhelmed and not sure where you're going."

"Close your eyes…Really feel what is going on in your body."

I did as I was told and searched for some mysterious feeling that had eluded me all these years.

"Would you say you are frightened? Do you perceive impending danger?"

"No. I'd maybe say I was exhausted—apprehensive about the future."

"Is that uncertainty about something that is happening right now, or what might happen later in the day or next week?"

"Later in the day," I responded. "I keep wondering what you'll come up with next."

The swami smiled. "Can you see a difference between the worries you've had during the past month and the exact concerns you have for this very moment?"

I nodded again. "But I have to deal with those problems sometime."

"Most people's lives are full of problems, David. I have a few of them myself here at the ashram…But what I want you to focus on while you are here are the problems you have on your plate this very moment. If you can, pinpoint one, then come up with a solution for it. When you are totally preoccupied with a disaster that could happen in ten minutes, or ten hours, or ten years, there's no room for anything new to come into your life. You have to make space for the solution."

The swami slowly rose from the chair and motioned for me to follow her. "Come into the other room with me."

I followed hesitantly, wondering what she had in mind for me. She pushed open the door to the room where we had first practised mantra together and waved me in.

"Stand here, David. Look in the mirror and tell me what you see."

She stood just inside the door looking not at me, but at the mirror. I stooped and stared at my reflection, feeling decidedly uneasy at the unexpected attention. What was she getting at, anyway?

"I don't understand," I muttered lamely. "I'm looking at my reflection—like you told me to."

"And what do you see?"

"Well," I began awkwardly, "I have a big nose."

The swami's face remained expressionless.

"I've got blue eyes…moles all over my face—a big one on the end of my nose that I've always hated. I've got long hair—should have gotten a haircut. Starting to see a wrinkle on my forehead."

I stopped and continued to study the image in the mirror. Swami Radha waited silently at the door. Was I missing something? What in the world was she trying to get at? I simply stood there, stubbornly staring at the dark brown eyes that reflected back at me from the mirror. It was several minutes later that she spoke.

"Is that all you see?"

"All I can think of."

"You described a lot of features. I'm not sure other people see them as you do. But even if they do, what are those features saying?"

I stood rigidly staring at the mirror. "What do you mean, *saying*?" I sighed. This woman was one strange cookie. I inspected my face in frustration for a moment more, then squirmed and looked down at my feet.

"Your eyes," she prompted. "Tell me more about your eyes."

"They're blue...Ugh, I told you that already. Oh man...I don't know what you want."

My inquisitor peered relentlessly into the glass until I finally engaged her eyes once more.

"Your eyes are the windows to your soul, David. What are they saying right now? What emotions are you able to see?"

I looked at the image in the mirror again. I suddenly pictured one of the rats I'd been forced to handle in physiology class during my second year at the veterinary college. There it was in my eyes—the same look of dread that rat had portrayed as it dangled by its tail waiting for me to make the uncertain lunge to grasp it by the scruff of the neck. And there, too, was the apprehension that I myself felt, anticipating the penetration of those sharp yellow teeth into the tender meat of my finger.

"Fear," I replied. "Exhaustion...anguish...remorse."

The swami turned and left the room. Before I could follow after her, she returned with a pad of lined foolscap. Drawing a line down the centre of the page, she wrote the word "Like" in the upper left corner and "Dislike" in the upper right.

"I want you to tell me all the things you like about yourself on this side, David. All the things you don't like on the other. Give me everything, not just the superficial things. Press hard. You are making a carbon copy for yourself."

She handed me the paper and pen, turned on her heel, and left the room. I studied my image in the mirror. What did I like about myself? Was there anything? I glanced at the pad and fumbled with the carbon paper that was sandwiched between the pages. *I like the colour of my eyes*, I began. *Most of the time, I like my height. I hate the moles all over my face—especially that ugly one on the end of my nose.* I sat for a moment pondering where to go from there. I didn't seem to have much trouble finding fault...It was much more of a chore to think of things that I did like about myself.

An hour later I emerged from the room. In the kitchen, Rita was pouring boiling water from the kettle into a teapot.

"Could you tell Swami Radha that I'm finished."

"Sure thing," she replied.

I returned to the room in the hallway and sat to look over the comments I had written. The page looked rather unbalanced with the half-dozen notations on the left side and a long list of criticisms spilling over to the back page on the right.

"Swami Radha will see you now," Rita said softly from the doorway.

The swami was seated in her overstuffed chair in the living room. Her feet were on a footstool. I waited for her to take a sip of her tea and return the cup to its saucer. "So you have finished," she acknowledged quietly.

I nodded and handed her the top copy of the document. She read it and set the sheet aside without comment.

"I have a list of questions that I want you to answer. I'd like for you to use a carbon with these as well."

I sat on the sofa and prepared my paper.

"What is ego?"

I jotted it down, then looked up at her blankly.

"What is your body?"

I made the notation but wondered at the silliness of the question.

"What is your soul?"

How was I to answer such esoteric questions?

"What is mind?" She waited while I caught up with my writing. "Define God…What comes to mind when we speak of the Divine?" The swami stared past me into the distance. "Give these questions some thought when you have time throughout the day, David. I've made arrangements for you to join the Hatha Yoga classes in the morning. They begin at seven o'clock in Saraswati Room. *Satsang* is a devotional service that we observe as a celebration of the day. It begins at eight every evening…It's held in Saraswati as well. For the rest of the afternoon you'll be doing karma yoga. If you see Ron, he'll assign a job to you."

"Karma yoga?" I asked. "What does that entail?"

"Have you noticed the people at work around the ashram?"

"Yes."

"They are performing selfless service. Karma yoga is the yoga of action without the desire for the fruits of the work. The goal of yoga is to become one with the Light. My guru, Swami Sivananda, used to say that selfless service was the way to achieve this. 'Selfless service will make you Divine,' he would often say. He told people to concentrate on that instead of intellectualizing on concepts like liberation.

"Just remember, David, that no work is too lowly to be done in Divine Mother's service, and none is too lowly for you to learn from. There are many things that you can learn from a weedy row of carrots, and often when people are asked to work in the kitchen, they think, *Oh, I am only in the kitchen.* Only? I learned some of my most important lessons in the kitchen. I did all the ashram cooking in the early days, and I did it on a stove with no heat controls. I started with all kinds of notions about the wonderful meals I was going to prepare, but the stove could handle only the simplest of cooking. Even then, I sometimes burned the food or didn't cook it through. I learned a lot about pride and letting go of results through my efforts in the kitchen."

The swami looked at me in a motherly fashion and paused.

"The idea of getting rewards for work is a trap that will swallow up the benefits of your efforts to be spiritual. Jesus said if you expect rewards on Earth for what you do, you may get them, but you can't then have rewards in heaven, too. When you work for the Divine, you don't get paid in dollars and cents. But if you learn to surrender, who is to say that isn't enough reward in itself?"

The swami took a sip of her tea, set her cup down, and then picked up the top page of her manuscript. I waited for more, but the look on her face suggested that our conversation was over.

I left Many Mansions in a total quandary. What an introduction to ashram life! I came looking for answers and got barraged with more questions. I needed relaxation and got new tasks to perform. Hell, if that was all I needed, I had enough jobs back in Creston to keep me busy for ten years. What long-term benefit could possibly accrue from spending the afternoon crawling around on my hands and knees in the ashram garden?

Mom and Dad had painfully drilled in the difference between a weed and a vegetable back in our garden in Casino. Did the ashram soil have some sort of mystical message encoded in it?

I was almost back to the bookstore when I found Ron outfitting a team for a woodcutting venture. The truck was already loaded with chainsaws and axes. Several karma yogis waited patiently in the cab. Three more sat on the wheel hubs in the back. I smiled. This day might just turn out better than I thought—I'd always gotten a big kick out of working in the bush. Swinging an axe or running a chainsaw just may be the ticket to boosting my morale. Right now, it would certainly beat weeding the garden. Maybe there was something to this karma yoga, after all.

"Hello, Ron."

"Hi, Dave…So are you finished with Swami Radha for the afternoon?"

"Yes. She's given me enough homework to keep me going into the wee hours, though."

Ron smiled. "Welcome to the ashram."

"Do you need a hand?" I asked. "Swami Radha has placed me in your capable hands for the afternoon."

"You can put those gas cans in the back, if you will."

I grabbed two gallon containers with *Mixed Gas* scrawled across the top of them and settled them in the back of the truck.

"Anything else?" I asked as he loaded another chainsaw.

"No, I think we're ready to go."

"Okay." I lifted my leg for the swing into the back of the truck.

"I've made arrangements for you to give Terrence a hand for the afternoon," Ron said casually.

"Terrence?"

"Yes…you'll find him over at Main House."

"The kitchen?" I stood with my mouth agape as Ron hopped in the vehicle and started the truck.

"Yes…just give a knock on the back door."

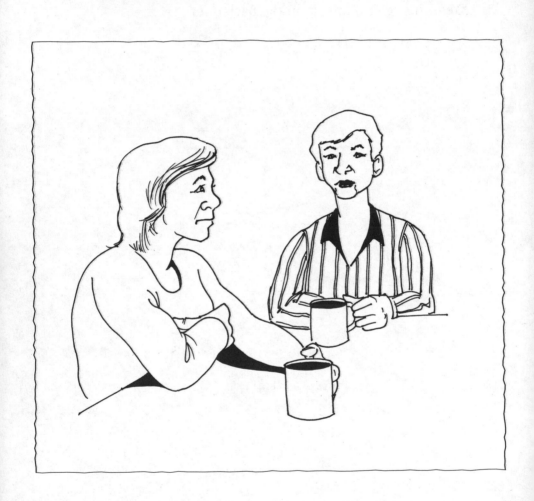

Tea with Tim

"Om namah sivaya, Om namah sivaya, Om…"

The pitch and tone of my lament varied as I wailed on. My voice cracked when I tried reaching the high note in the third element, but I trucked on as if it were meant to be. Tears welled as the foreign words of the mantra echoed in the room. I had been battling all morning to focus on the words and drive the other relentless, repetitive thoughts from my mind. I remembered what Swami Radha was trying to teach me: that so much of our time is spent in judgement. She had said, "Mantra helps one to focus attention and prevent the constant wandering of the mind."

"Om namah sivaya, Om namah…" Cory and I were back in Saskatoon struggling through a study session together. I closed my eyes and belted out another verse of the mantra. Suddenly, I saw Marcie being flung from our careening raft. I instinctively craned my neck as I watched her bobbing in the murky runoff waters of the Moyie River. I caught myself wandering and reluctantly returned to the mantra. I relished the simplicity of the words. I focused on their reverberation in the back of my throat; I prolonged the "Om-m-m" until my lips tickled from the vibration.

I cringed at the terrible grinding as John worked the stick of my transmission into third gear. In my mind's eye, Brian covered his head and dove for the back seat as the car careened toward the ditch. "Om namah…" Brian's face was chalk white as his lifeless form lay stretched in his coffin. The "Om" that exploded from my throat jolted me. *Oh God, how could you have killed him before I could see him again?*

I twitched, opened my eyes uneasily, ran my sleeve over my cheeks, and glanced at my watch. It was almost two o'clock—time for another session with Swami Radha. I closed my eyes and sat for a few moments focusing on the flow of my breath. I was possessed by an eerie calm. A little voice murmured that I was fine—I was in the right place at the right time.

I descended the sixty-seven wooden stairs to the road. I walked slowly, conscious of the crunch of the gravel beneath my feet. Taking a deep breath, I tried to place the earthy fragrance that hung on the breeze. Was it the smell of wet grass? I realized instinctively that at this time last week I never would have noticed it, never mind have tried to identify it.

I paused as a sprinkler finished its circuit in front of me, then passed on. The trail to Swami Radha's house led through the orchard past several rustic storage buildings. I nodded to Ron and a helper as the pair balanced the partially erected form for the wall of a new root cellar. The ashram was constantly expanding to fulfill the needs of the residents.

I found the swami in her garden seated at a wrought-iron table beneath an elaborate tentlike structure of nylon screening.

"Hello, David." Swami Radha looked up from a page of hand-scrawled notes that she had been studying. "Come in. Come in."

I opened the zipper and ducked into the tent. The swami pointed to a chair across from her.

"Sit down…Can I pour you some tea?"

I nodded and she filled the cup that was already set out across the table from her. She smiled at me as I settled stiffly into a chair that came halfway up my back.

"How are you today?"

"Better," I replied. "I still find myself welling up with tears constantly—but I definitely feel better."

"Have you looked to the source of them?" Her steely eyes engaged mine over the rim of her teacup. I looked toward the orchard and struggled with my composure.

"I'm not sure what you mean," I said.

"Are they tears of grief, of bitterness, of healing?" She shuffled the papers on her lap, then looked at me intently. "Or are these tears of self-pity?" Her voice was almost deadpan.

"Does it matter?" I struggled with the import of the words she had used. "Self-pity" sounded so indulgent. What right had she to question my motives, anyway? She would feel differently if Brian had been close to her.

"What do you think?" She gazed at me as I squirmed on the edge of my chair. Several uncomfortable minutes passed in silence as I waited for her to say more. My guru slowly raised her cup and took a sip of tea. Her eyes never left my face.

"I guess it does," I finally admitted.

"Why?" she asked softly, still surveying my face.

I wilted. Why didn't she just tell me why it mattered? I might have known that she wasn't about to give something away. Questions—always questions, questions, and more questions. Couldn't she understand that I had come back here looking for answers, not more questions?

I sat in stony silence. Not a wheel turned. A rebellious child, I suddenly didn't want to be here.

"Is there a pattern, David?"

"A pattern?"

"Are there any similarities between this and other things that have happened in your life?"

"No one close to me has ever died before."

"And no one close to you has ever let you down, ever disappointed you?"

"I never said that."

"How do you react when people let you down? When they disappoint you? When they don't live up to your expectations?"

I thought about Marcie and Cory. How did that relate? Was I grieving a loss there, too? Can you grieve the loss of something you never really had?

"Can you find a pattern, David—a way that your mind responds to any insult or any attack upon the status quo?"

I sat staring off into space—not thinking of a pattern, not thinking at all. Was that a pattern in itself? Did I often shut down when faced with a question I'd rather not face?

"One of the fundamentals of yoga is looking at what you are and who you are. A psychologist focuses on having a patient relive the past and then deal with the emotions that surface. A yogi is more interested in searching out how you get to where you are. If you truly understand your own motives and patterns of reaction, then you can keep from repeating the same mistakes over and over again."

"I find that I just want to be alone," I whispered fervently, "to do what I need to do and get on with the day. It would be a lot simpler if I didn't have to go off to meaningless jobs working with people I'm never going to see again."

Swami Radha took a sip of her tea. Her eyes were focused on my face.

"David…David, can't you see how much you can learn about yourself by working with others? By coming into contact with people in an environment like the ashram, we can often learn what our trigger points are. Conflicts with other people are an ideal starting point for working out conflicts within ourselves.

"You've been wandering around the grounds lost in your own world. Although many saints have gained enlightenment by seeking solitude, opening yourself up to other humans on the path and truly listening to what they have to say can dramatically speed your journey. Understand what others feel; really watch what you feel toward them. By letting yourself feel their pain and allowing them to see your fears, you can both grow and understand the meaning of compassion.

"Go with the process—accept that there may be something you don't understand that could have merit. Take a few steps into the darkened room and accept that you may well find a candle and the match to light it. Surrendering to Divine guidance can be exactly that. I expect to say a few words about surrender at *satsang* tonight."

As I was getting up to leave, she said, "What do you want from life right now, David? If you could have anything in the whole world, what would you want? I want you to take some time and ask yourself that question. Write it all down so you know, and sort through your feelings. How can you make it to your goals when you can't tell me what they are?"

Later I again sat with Swami Radha, but twenty other people had joined us for the evening devotional. One of the participants, a young man named Ralph, who still wore the same dusty clothes he had worn all day in the garden, was confronting the swami. Seated with his long legs in a half lotus position, he leaned forward from the waist to emphasize his point. His jaw jutted forward. He looked around him at the others in the circle and shrugged his disbelief.

"You speak of surrender as if it's something positive," Ralph challenged. "How can that be? What has ever been accomplished by giving up?"

He was voicing my own concern. The word "surrender" was being bantered about at this place as if it were a solution for everything. The swami's face remained contemplative. Focusing her gaze on Ralph, she nodded thoughtfully.

"We in the West tend to attach all sorts of negative connotations to the word 'surrender.' To many, it implies defeat—giving up something that we really want to hold onto. One would think that it was the lazy thing to do, the cowardly thing. Far from it. Surrender can be a life quest—a mission statement for many lifetimes. It doesn't mean that you have to be passive and tolerate any situation you happen to be in. I am not telling you to do nothing to change your circumstances or to quit making plans for real change. To be able to surrender and wear the cloak of humility is a very important requirement in the practice of yoga."

She paused and we all waited expectantly for her to carry on.

"What do we surrender on the altar of the Divine?" she finally asked. "The list is legion...pride, arrogance, lust, self-pity." She looked beyond Ralph and gazed right at me.

"When I first went to India to study under Swami Sivananda, he drew a line down the centre of a page and asked me to write down all the things I liked about myself, all the things I disliked. I came back and presented a document with a long line of dislikes and only a few likes...He glanced at it and threw it back at me. 'False pride,' he said."

I squirmed in my seat as she continued.

"Surrender comes into every aspect of the spiritual life...What can be more difficult than to surrender our judgements—our judgements of both ourselves and of others? When was the last time you were critical of someone you worked with here at the ashram?"

I immediately thought of my interaction with Jocelyn in the garden that afternoon. Man, I had been a total idiot in dealing with her. What difference did it make to me whether the woman actually accomplished something or just sat around in the sun all day? What right had I to be her judge?

"When was the last time you were critical of yourself and passed judgement?"

I winced as I realized that I was busily doing that right now. I closed my eyes and tried to focus on every word that came out of the swami's mouth.

"Our world abounds with beauty. How precious the bounties that have been bestowed upon each and every one of us...But how often do we stand surrounded by our bounties, here in all this natural splendour, and pay it no heed? How often are we given gifts from the Divine that we don't recognize and don't give thanks for because we are intent on them happening exactly the way we want them to happen?"

Making eye contact with one person after the other, she seemed to communicate with each in turn.

"We are also talking about the surrender of opinions and preconceived ideas…When was the last time you really listened to a friend? Think back to the moment."

She paused as we all tried to remember. "Were you able to surrender your desire to express your own opinion—to keep from trying to direct his or her train of thought to your own way of thinking? How can you possibly listen—and I mean truly listen, without first surrendering the desire to be heard, then the desire to sell your point of view? When you listen to your friends, you owe it to them and yourself to do so with no hidden agenda and no preconceived ideas. You surrender your point of view."

I thought back to my first session with Swami Radha—how she had sat in silence for hours. Not once had she made any attempt to direct my diatribe.

"Once you have learned to listen to another person, you can apply a similar approach to listening to yourself. Only when you have learned to relax the body and surrender the constant flow of thoughts and movements can you prepare for total relaxation—surrender to the flow of breath into the body and out of it. Flowing with the breath of life will still the mind and allow intuition to flow like never before."

She paused again. Her breaths were long and deliberate. Silence pervaded the room. I closed my eyes and focused on the flow of air at the tip of my nostrils. When she began speaking again, it was as if she were at the end of a long tunnel.

"In every person's life are going to be times of plenty. There will also be cycles when failure or perceived failure will lead to things withering and fading away. If you cling to those physical things, if you cling to the past, you are guaranteed to suffer and hold back the inevitable period of regeneration that will follow if you only allow it to happen. Failure is often the only way to make new room in your life; without it you would not grow. Look around this room."

We each surveyed the room, taking in the persona of one person after the other. My focus fell on Tim Brady. He was the middle-aged man I had noticed weeding the garden on my arrival. Although he smiled from time to time, he rarely said anything. What was it about him that bothered me so?

"Really look at the people next to you," Swami Radha entreated. "You know something of their stories, and they know something about you."

I continued to stare at Tim's profile, trying to understand why he made me uncomfortable.

"Would any of us have turned to the spiritual path unless we had failed or unless our successes suddenly seemed to have lost meaning? All things that man builds are destined to decay. As long as you derive your self-worth from your worldly possessions, from your achievements, from your position in the community, you are destined to know pain. All these things will pass away...All these things will change. Only by surrendering to those inevitable changes can you know peace."

The swami closed her eyes and again sat in silence. Five minutes later she rose and headed for the exit. The class was over. I stacked my stool by the door and wandered out into the evening air.

I was in a pensive mood. For the last two weeks I had been struggling with the realization that I was constantly judging—judging situations as good or bad, judging points of view as right or wrong, judging people on superficial merits as being useful members of society or hopeless wastes of human skin.

I had worked diligently pointing out these transgressions to myself. Identifying them as they occurred, I tried to stomp them out. It wasn't until Swami Radha asked her question about being critical of oneself that I realized the truth. I had not stopped judging at all—just shifted the focus slightly away from others and onto me and my own imperfections.

I suddenly felt tired of this—all of this. I didn't want to spend the rest of my life riding herd on the thoughts that I was or wasn't allowed to express. Weeding the ashram garden was a breeze when compared with weeding my mind. At least when I pulled a weed from the ground, I could watch it wither in the sun. But I'd weed out a thought, and ten seconds later it would be back—with a dozen more just like it.

I walked to the end of the sidewalk. Stepping onto the grass, I waited for the others to pass. I looked up at the stars. Swami Radha was right—how could we take something like this for granted? How could a man look up at the night sky and be unmoved by its majesty?

I suddenly wanted to escape all that man had created—the lamp over my head, the concrete underfoot. I wanted to be alone with nature. I descended the stairs almost dreamily—paying attention to where my feet were landing, but looking up at the night sky as well. The moon was almost full, and its light reflected with a shimmering incandescence from the surface of the lake. At that moment, I was part of everything that ever was—everything was a part of me.

I gravitated toward the lake. The crunch of dry grass beneath my sandals gave way to the dull grinding of stones. I extended my arms into the air as I moved forward—felt the breeze gently ruffle my hair. The air smelled so fresh—moist and clean. I sat on the huge moulded block of stone, my throne, and ran my hand over its weathered exterior. Still warm from a day in the hot sun, it was so smooth and worn. Would I have as much character when all my rough edges had been knocked off? Would I exude quality, longevity, resilience—the way the granite beneath me now did? Tonight, anything was possible.

How different I felt from the first day I had arrived. It would be stretching it to think that I had become the person I wanted to be—the person I knew lay deep within. But I had a strange sense of peace that had seemed so unattainable just two weeks before. What had changed?

I sat on the rock drinking in the noisy silence of the night. The rumble of the stream as water tumbled to the lake at the corner of the ashram property, the soft wooing of a nighthawk somewhere in the distance, a raised voice from the plateau above—all blended into the moment. I opened my eyes and shared the view with my other senses. The surface of the water blended into the darkness of the opposite shore, where lights shone from a dozen cottages. A red light flashed from the hydro tower. Row after row of purple mountains blended with one another as they faded into the distant sky.

How far away the trauma in my life now seemed. I had hardly thought about the office in the last several days. Once in meditation, I had seen Cory working with a herd of cows. I wondered how he was managing. I sat for half an hour in contemplation. For a few moments I was granite as I became one with my stone throne.

It was getting late. I had gotten into the routine of waking around six and waiting my turn for the community bathroom. By seven, when Hatha Yoga started, I was showered and ready to face the day.

The prayer room was dark as I ascended the earthen steps to Main House. The lights were still on in the dining hall, and I found myself drawn in that direction. I glanced through the window. The room was unoccupied. I would just slip in for a cup of tea. Somehow I still wasn't ready for sleep.

The screen door banged behind me. The sound that the rolling latch mechanism made on the door reminded me of Grandpa's place, and for just a moment I was back there on the hill overlooking the Creston Valley.

I ventured to the far end of the room and grabbed the kettle. It was still half full from its previous user, and still too hot to comfortably handle. I plugged it in. As the water started grumbling, I grabbed a cup and surveyed the jars of herbs. I considered a chamomile and lemon grass combination, but settled on a commercial packet labelled cran-apple cinnamon. I had already poured the boiling water into my cup when the screen door opened. I looked up from my steaming concoction.

Damn…it was Tim Brady. He moved decisively across the room and plunked himself down on the end of my bench before I could mobilize myself into evacuation.

"Good evening," he said cheerfully.

"Good evening," I responded. I glanced furtively at the bench behind him. It was crammed tight to the wall. I sighed. There were three ways out: I could crawl under the table, step onto the table, or ask him to get up to let me go.

"Trouble sleeping, too?" he asked.

"Just on my way up to give it a shot," I muttered. I played with my spoon in my mug. Trapping the teabag against the side of the cup, I watched the rich, reddish-brown liquid diffuse into the water.

"How are things going?"

"Better," I responded.

An uncomfortable silence prevailed as I sipped at the tart, steaming liquid. He grabbed a mug and a packet of Blue Ribbon tea. After tearing open the paper envelope, he sat for a moment. I passed him the kettle.

"Thank you," he muttered.

"Welcome."

I began wishing that I had just used the water directly from the kettle on arrival. If I had done that, I could have just gulped the tea down and excused myself. As it was, my progress was pathetically slow. I could swallow it only one tiny blistering sip at a time.

I perused the room, pausing on a picture of Swami Radha seated on a tiger skin next to a jovial-looking man that I knew to be Swami Sivananda. I wondered if meditating every day on a tiger skin would make a difference in my ability to concentrate.

"You don't like me, do you?"

Tim's question caught me off guard. Thoughts of the tiger skin disappeared. I flushed and looked at him. My first instinct was to deny his accusation and ask him why he thought that…but I was here at the ashram in search of truth.

"Not particularly," I replied. I began fishing around in my mug with my spoon.

"Can you tell me why?" He stared straight at me, his blue-green eyes focused on mine.

"Don't know. Does it matter?"

"Don't you think it should matter? We're both here to try and sort out our reactions in the real world. Maybe trying to understand your feelings toward me will help you shed light on an existing problem out there."

I stared into my cup. This was the last thing I needed right now. Why couldn't he just mind his own bloody business and leave me alone? We sat in silence for several minutes, sipping idly at our tea. I tried to take a large swallow and lowered my mug so quickly that I spilled some on the table. Damn—I had burned the roof of my mouth.

Tim reached over to a dispenser and passed me a napkin. In doing so, he looked directly at me. The expression on his lean face was gentle—with not a hint of malice. "I wouldn't push this, but Swami Radha asked me to speak with you…She suggested that we have a lot to learn from one another. I'm not sure what it is, but over the last few months I've come to value her opinion."

I felt much as I always had when asked to stand up in class and give my opinion. God, I hated to be singled out when I wasn't ready for it. It was bad enough when I had a week to sort things out—to formulate my opinion. Were my ears as red as I thought they were? If so, I had already dug myself a very big psychological deficit. I sat stubbornly in silence.

"Was it something I said?" he finally asked.

For several minutes, I didn't even try to formulate a response. I started talking without having considered what I was going to say.

"I guess I respect people for what they do. I can sort of see why some of the younger guys are here. A lot of them are kids trying to figure out where they want to go…but you…"

His eyes focused on my face. I fished uncomfortably for a way of softening my message—of cushioning my truth.

"All my friends are people with ambition—people with goals. Look at you, an overgrown hippie crawling around weeding the garden on your hands and knees. Hell, if you haven't found something that you can do in the real world by now, when will you?"

I paused, avoiding his eyes. "I guess by the time I get to be your age, I want a life of my own—something to show for the time that I've spent." I took a healthy sip of the tea. It was finally cooling off enough for me to drink it and get out of here.

Tim gazed at the screen door as if expecting it to provide an answer.

"Things are not always as they seem," he said. "I guess when I was your age, my thinking was a lot like yours. Everything I did was to accomplish a goal. I went to university and scraped for top marks. If I didn't get A, I'd go to my prof and challenge his marking. I needed the best marks I could get to be admitted to architectural college."

He looked back at me. He had my attention.

"I graduated top in my class and worked like a hound to establish my reputation. I wanted lots of money and all the things that money could buy. It was always my goal to be a millionaire. I was just completing a large office building in Calgary when my accountant told me that, on paper, I had hit the mark."

He paused. When he began again, he looked somehow very sad.

"You know, there were no tickertape parades…no banners flying. One day I didn't know I was worth a million, the next I did."

He nursed his tea and continued to stare at the exit. Neither of us spoke for a while. I drained my mug, set it down, and gazed at the same door as if resolution to our problems lay just beyond.

301

"A few months ago," he said in a quiet voice, "my wife packed up the kids and left me...I guess I'm here regrouping."

We sat in silence for several more minutes before he stood, placed his cup in the sink, and left. The screen door slammed and I was once more alone.

Four-Letter Word

I awoke to the sound of my neighbour rustling around in the adjoining room. Those cedar walls may have been rustic, but they were a long way from being soundproof. I scurried across the hall to the bathroom juggling my soap, towel, shaving kit, and water glass. Rousting myself at six every morning had become part of ashram routine—sleeping in often cost me the opportunity to shower.

Rubbing the steam from the upper edge of the mirror, I scraped at my face with a razor that had seen far too much use. I concentrated on an area of my chin where a scraggy patch of resilient hair resisted my efforts. It was definitely time for a new razor.

I wiped a few gobs of shaving cream from my face and went though my new ritual. Taking a deep breath, I stared into the mirror, intent on following the swami's instructions. Would I ever be able to fall in love with this face? As always, my moles were my first focus. A small nick on the edge of the one on my right cheek was still oozing blood. I studied the blemishes one after another, wondering how much different I'd have looked if I hadn't been cursed with their presence. How I hated the one on the end of my nose. Every time I focused on it, I was back in the schoolyard hearing, "Here comes Beauty Pimples!"

My mind flashed to an uncomfortable moment with a client only a short while before Cory and Marcie's arrival. Betty Wilde had been in with her cat, Felix, for his vaccination. Her four-year-old son, Justin, had stared with fascination at my face. To his mother's annoyance, he repeatedly yanked on her sleeve and asked

303

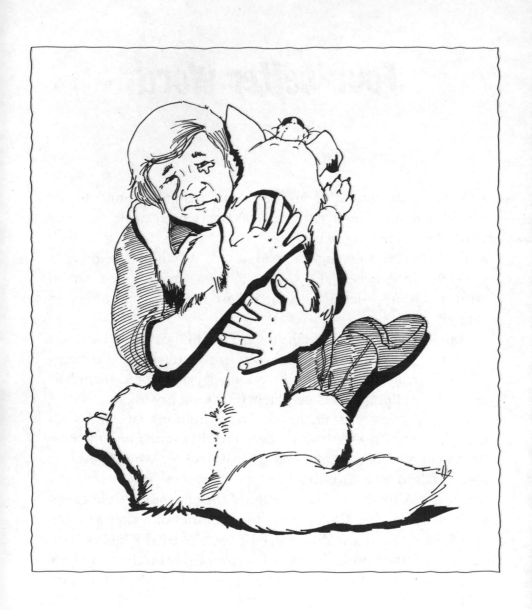

in a hushed tone, "What's that funny thing on the man's nose, Mommy?" I finally halted my examination of the cat and explained to the boy that it was a mole and that I thought it was pretty funny-looking, too.

I allowed my focus to wander around my face. Hair hung in my eyes and the tips of my ears were barely visible—I was definitely overdue for a trip to Manell's. Wouldn't Doris love to take the clippers to that crop? I could hear her mock threatening tone. I would miss her terribly.

As always, my focus narrowed to the eyes. I was intent on softening around their perimeter for that oh-so-difficult exercise—the wielding of the four-letter word. *I love you,* I mouthed. Repeating it half a dozen times, I tried to convince myself that I really meant it. I abandoned the effort as I had every morning for the past fifteen days. I brushed my teeth and hopped into the shower.

I arrived at the Hatha Yoga class early and rolled out a rubber mat in a corner where I would have a good view of the instructor without being viewed by the other participants. Two weeks ago, I had felt foolish attempting even the simplest of poses, but at Swami Radha's urging, I had persisted. Little by little, my clunky body was becoming more responsive and, yes, even more flexible.

This was the second day of an intensive yoga workshop—the entire time would be spent doing poses and reflecting upon life questions. The day before, we had gone through structural postures like the Mountain, Triangle, Shoulder Stand, and Forward Bend. Many of the people in this class had been practising these same *asanas* for decades. It was intimidating always being the beginner, but I had resigned myself to accepting my body for what it was at the present.

After a series of warm-ups and flexibility poses, we worked with tool postures—the Plough and the Bow—both of which I managed to fake well enough that by lunchtime I was feeling part of the group.

Whether it was the five hours of exercise, or the fact that I had eaten little for breakfast, I was starving when I headed down the hill to Main House. I loaded my plate with several different salads. Today there were two hot dishes—one of lentils and another of baked beans. I added several heaping ladles of each. Still not used to the fact that the diet here was mostly vegetarian, I'd have given anything to be tackling a nice steak or even a juicy hamburger.

Over the lunch break I became cognizant of the constant rumble in my stomach. I should have known better than to pig out on baked beans. I soon found myself perched on my familiar stone throne on the beach, where I could break wind in solitude.

As usual, we began the afternoon session with a relaxation pose called Rejuvenation. With our arms at our sides, we moved our bodies back and forth and slowly wilted forward until our heads were swinging as low as our bodies would permit. I managed to unobtrusively dispose of a bit of gas during this exercise. Judging from the aroma of the room when we moved on to the Alexander Shoulder Stretch, I wasn't the only one.

"We'll do some Rock and Rolls to limber up our spine," our instructor counselled.

I moved to the foot of my mat and balanced on the base of my spine, slowly rotating my body. Moving my hands to my ankles, I began rocking gently back and forth, starting at a sitting position and ending with my weight on my shoulders and the back of my neck. I had performed the movement a few times. It was when I arched back with my butt in the air that it happened—an explosive burst that would have satisfied any adolescent fantasy.

I heard titters around the room, but before I had reached the upright position I was answered from first one side of the room, then the other. The warm-up faded as one after the other of the participants collapsed in laughter. Someone would have to talk to the cook about the menu for intensive Hatha days.

After the class settled down, our instructor read from material on the Tree posture that Swami Radha had prepared. She demonstrated the pose and selected a portion of the passage to reread.

Finally, she presented us with a series of questions to take into the pose. "Where have my roots spread? Where do they get their nourishment? Which roots are mine, and which belong to a neighbouring tree? What competes with my roots for nourishment?" My mind was actively contemplating the questions long before I tried the position. Did I even have roots? Would I just wither and die without my practice?

In front of me, the slender blonde schoolteacher from Ontario gracefully lifted her right foot and placed it on the inside of her left thigh. With her knee at a perfect right angle to her body, she stretched her arms to her side, then easily brought them together over her head. Holding that position for a full minute, she opened her arms to shoulder-width—she was a tree spreading her branches to the sun.

Glancing around the room at all the one-legged trees, at all the branches basking in the sunlight, I prayed that if this tree fell in the forest, it wouldn't crush another on the way down. After all, when we spread our arms at the same time, our hands would be likely to touch those of our neighbour.

I stood on my left foot with my arms at my side and tentatively lifted my right. I bent my leg and shakily brought the flat of my foot toward my opposite knee. I wobbled and toppled to the side.

"Remember the balance between strength and flexibility," our instructor chimed. "The oak wants to be strong but needs to bend in the wind. The willow needs flexibility, but still must have the strength to support itself."

My friend from Ontario had already held her pose for several minutes. She lowered her arms ever so slowly to her side, and her raised foot to the floor. Standing rock-still in the Mountain pose, she stared out the window.

I stood on one foot and lifted the other off the ground. Holding this position for thirty seconds, I closed my eyes and pictured my gangly frame balanced and poised. I lifted my leg higher and turned my knee to the side. For several moments my tree stood strong and straight. I held my arms at right angles to my body. Slowly I raised them over my head. I wobbled and brought them back to shoulder height. Too late—the old snag came crashing to the ground. This was harder than it looked.

The woman in front of me lifted her left foot elegantly and placed it on her right thigh. Ever so slowly her arms drifted first to the peak position and then to the open arms position. I shook my head in disgust. Maybe I should try balancing on my other foot, too. I raised my leg and struggled to a standstill. The moment I lifted my arms, all was lost.

For ten minutes I battled to master the pose. The space around me grew as my fellow participants gave me more room to dance around. Why in the world could I not stand on one foot? I was ready to give up in frustration and simply visualize the pose when our instructor once more read out the questions. "Where have my roots spread? Where do they get their nourishment? Which are mine, and which belong to a neighbouring tree? What competes with my roots for nourishment?"

Changing my position so that I could gaze out the window, I focused on a stately fir that stood just over the brow of the hill. Straight and tall, it was swaying gently back and forth in the wind. I lifted my right foot and placed it on my left thigh. My arms swung up to shoulder height and peaked over my head. I opened my arms and stood steadily for several minutes, focusing on the question: Where do I get my nourishment?

It was as though my inner voice were screaming the answer out loud. *From my work! I get my sustenance from helping others, from doing my job as well as I can do it.*

With a sudden feeling of well-being, I lowered my arms, placed both feet on the floor, and stood transfixed, my eyes on the stately fir that had taught me to be a tree. As if I had been doing the pose for decades, I reversed my stance and held the posture on the other foot without so much as a waver.

I was going home…I was going back to reclaim what would be

my salvation. I was going back to Lug and Doris and Creston and my clients. I was going back to my farm. It was time.

Swami Radha smiled and gave me a knowing look when I informed her of my decision to leave. "You're a great veterinarian and a caring man, David. I can't think of a better place for you to learn about yourself than in daily service to your clients."

After a long discussion about easing myself back into practice, she convinced me to stay until after the rose ceremony. "You need closure in your dealings with Marcie and Cory. You have to let go of your regrets about Brian. Maybe the rose ceremony will give that to you."

The next afternoon I joined the others who were taking part in the ceremony. From the vase of roses offered to each of us, I selected a beautiful red bloom—what a shame to sacrifice it. Standing before the altar, I plucked the silky petals from the flower one at a time and dropped them into a crystal bowl filled with water. With each petal deposited, I recited a pair of opposites— love and hate, honesty and deception, selfishness and selflessness, anger and compassion, greed and generosity.

With each opposite, a significant face or action flashed through my mind. Sometimes I remembered a simple act of kindness, and a smiling face came into view. Sometimes I remembered something I was less than proud of, and I would see the frowning face of someone for whom I had caused pain or disappointment.

When everyone had presented their rose to the water, Swami Radha instructed us to spend the evening listing all of our grudges and resentments. We were to bring them to the beach the following morning for the conclusion of the ceremony.

I spent hours digging through my memory banks rousting out every feeling of animosity that lurked within me. It was hard to believe that twenty years after some kid had tormented me on the school playground, I could still be wasting energy fretting over it. I wrote until I had recorded even the most innocuous event, and slept deeply for the remaining few hours of the night.

On my last morning, I stood before the bonfire on the beach and threw my list of regrets into the flames. As it turned to ashes, I felt a strange relief, as if a tremendous weight had been hefted from my shoulders.

Swami Radha was right. The rose ceremony provided a form of closure to a lot of soul-searching. I had come to realize over my weeks at the ashram that my problems with Marcie and Cory had in fact been my problems, and that no matter how I justified my feelings toward them, the only person who was suffering as a result was me. Coming to an esoteric understanding of that was one thing—physically dealing with it was another.

I spent the afternoon at Mom and Dad's place in Riondel. Lug just about tied himself in a knot doing circles when I showed up at the house. Whenever I moved from one room to the next, the poor dog was there on my heels. I called Cory to make arrangements to meet with him later in the day—I was primed to rebuild the life that I had limped away from.

On the way to Creston, I turned in at the ashram and drove down the lane to Many Mansions. Swami Radha came to the door to say her farewell. After chatting for a moment, I gave her a hug and turned to leave.

"How goes the love affair?" she asked. Her dark eyes seemed to pierce me. "Are you still practising twice a day with the mirror?"

I nodded. "Can't say that I'm madly in love yet, though."

She smiled. "All is Light, David. Fall in love with the Light."

I shrugged and smiled meekly.

"Is that your dog in the car?"

"Yeah." Lug sat with his nose to the window, watching my every move. "He's not big on letting me out of his sight today. He likes Gramps a lot, but he doesn't want me to leave him behind again."

"He's a bright-looking dog…You must really love him."

"Yeah, he's quite a character."

"Why don't you give him a big hug for me...Tell him that you love him."

I flushed. "Well, I better get going. Thank you for everything."

I could feel her eyes on me as I slid onto the seat; I had a strange compulsion to do as she'd asked. Was she willing me to carry out her prescription? Lug leaned over and licked my cheek. I rumpled his ears and started the engine. Waving to the swami, I drove down the lane.

As I negotiated the sharp corners of Highway 3A, I fondled the small bottle of rosewater. This little sample, another jar containing some ashes, and a round stone from the beach were the only physical mementos of an experience I'd never forget.

I parked behind the clinic and walked up the side stairs. Lug thundered ahead of me, delighted to be home. I unlocked the door and walked in, leaving my suitcase on the landing. Surveying the apartment, I drank in the splendour.

The poster that a friend had given me to cover the hole I had punched in the wall still proclaimed: *Yea, though I walk through the valley of the shadow of death, I fear no evil, for I am the meanest son of a bitch in the valley.* The hole Shirley had burned in the carpet when she dropped the pressure cooker was still covered by the same red mat.

Nothing had changed, yet somehow everything looked different. I dug into my pocket for my souvenirs and lined them up on the table—my container of rosewater, the ashes, and my smooth, rounded stone. I removed the lid from the jar of ashes and rubbed some of the gritty powder between my fingertips.

Dust—nothing but dust—that's how my resentments would remain. I headed downstairs. It was time to talk to Cory. I found him in the lab making notations on a pet record. He flushed when he saw me. He wasn't looking forward to this meeting any more than I was.

"Hello, Cory."

"Hello," he answered tersely.

"How have things been going?"

"Good. We've been busy."

I nodded and stood studying his face for a moment. Swami Radha's words flashed through my mind: *To the degree that you can let go of your resentments and your grudges, you will be set free.*

"We have to come to some sort of resolution here," I said quietly.

He nodded.

"I'm coming back, Cory…For the time being, this is where I belong."

He looked away from me and scratched a few more notes on the card.

"I'll finish out the day," he said.

"Okay."

I ascended the stairs to my apartment and went directly to the bathroom. I stared into the mirror with an intensity that I had never seen before. Relaxing my features completely, I focused on my eyes. I paid little heed to the big nose that had distracted me on many other occasions, no attention to the mole that had so occupied my attention. I saw only the eyes.

"Show me compassion," I said in a quiet voice.

I stared at my eyes until I was convinced that they were the most compassionate eyes I had ever looked upon.

"Show me love."

My facial features softened even more. I studied myself without the slightest movement until my eyes began to burn. I blinked and returned to my task.

"I love you," I said hesitantly. The doubt had vanished. There was no question that the words had come directly from my heart. I stared into my eyes until I was totally lost in them—until there was nothing but Light looking at Light. I smiled.

"I love you," I repeated emphatically.

In a state of euphoria, I bounded into the kitchen. Lug stood there looking up at me, tail wagging. I threw myself on my knees and looked into his big brown knowing eyes.

"I love you," I blurted, throwing my arms around him. I buried my face in the nape of his neck and wept unabashedly, my tears soaking into his fur.

"Oh, Lug, I love you so much."

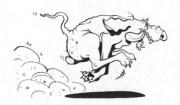